CONTENTS

Disclaimer Notice:

Chapter One

ESSENTIALS ABOUT THE PROGRAM

*W*ant to lose weight and still enjoy all your favorite foods? Then attempt on the Weight loss Freestyle Program. In this chapter, you will learn everything about Weight loss and how you can get started.

Advantages and Disadvantages of the Weight loss Diet

Weight loss is a widely popular and successful weight-loss program that has helped millions of people around the globe. But that doesn't necessarily mean it's right for everyone. It's essential you take a look at all the advantages and disadvantages of the Weight loss program before you commit.

Advantages of Weight loss

Here are some reasons why the diet plan may be the best route to help you lose weight.

- **No restrictions on food:** There is no official list of foods to avoid on Weight loss like you'll see on other diets. Instead, you track SmartPoints and garner FitPoints. The point system encourages you to eat more healthy foods such as fruits and vegetables while also enjoying your favorite sweets occasionally.
- **Nutritional value tips, cooking advice, recipes, and lifestyle changes are offered:** When you attend Weight loss meetings, meeting leaders is inclined to share effective

nutritional advice with participants, for example, discussing the importance of adding more vegetables, healthy fats, low-fat dairy, reduced sugar, and drinking plenty of water to your diet.

- **The program is eligible for kids:** Some Weight loss locations hold meetings open for children. Teens as young as 13-years-old can participate in the Weight loss program if they have physician approval.
- **Slow and steady weight loss:** If you choose to commit to this program, you can expect to lose 1 to 2 pounds per week. You might lose even more when you first begin. Losing weight at a slow and steady rate makes weight loss more stable.
- **The program encourages portion control:** In order to keep track and record your SmartPoints you will need to measure your portions and serving sizes. Being able to control your portions will benefit you beyond Weight loss.
- **The program encourages exercise:** The Weight loss program encourages daily exercise which earns you FitPoints. Earning FitPoints will balance out your food intake.
- **You will cook at home:** You are more likely to eat healthy foods if you prepare them yourself at home. Weight loss offers recipes using your Instant Pot to help you learn how to prepare healthy meals.

Disadvantages of Weight loss

While Weight loss is a perfect solution for many to lose weight, it may not be appropriate for you. Take a look at the disadvantages of the Weight loss program.

- **Weight loss can be pricey:** The monthly cost for joining the Weight loss program will vary based on the level you choose, but if you have a substantial amount of weight to lose, the investment may be costly.
- **Group meetings aren't for everyone:** Some people prefer to keep their personal health and weight loss information private. You are not required to talk at Weight loss meetings. But Weight loss meetings are what makes the program special. However, if you prefer to avoid meetings, there are other options.
- **Weekly weigh-ins are a must:** Weighing yourself once a

week to track your progress on the Weight loss program is a requirement. For some participants, this can be uncomfortable. For others, it keeps them motivated.

- **Weekly progress may discourage you:** Weekly progress checks can vary. Some weeks you will lose little weight. Sometimes you may even gain weight, even if you're doing everything right. This can discourage you from remaining in the program.
- **Keeping track of SmartPoints:** Keeping track of all the SmartPoints can be tedious and time-consuming.
- **Freedom to eat:** The Weight loss diet don't have any restrictions and you can eat almost anything you want. This freedom to eat anything you want can be too tempting. For some participants, diets that offer strict eating guidelines prove more effective.

Key Principles of Successful Weight loss and How It Works

Weight loss is an effective program because it's not really a diet. There are no specific restrictions on food intake, you just pay careful attention to portion sizes and keep track of SmartPoints.

Weight loss is less strict than many other diets – but the results are still promising, with participants able to lose up to 2- 4 pounds per week. This program still follows the three key principles: **Keep track of what you eat using SmartPoints, make healthy habits, and join a support group.**

Joining Weight loss, you learn how to calculate the number of Smart-Points to achieve your health and weight loss goals. Your daily and weekly SmartPoints allowance will be different depending on each person's status. After you are given a personalized SmartPoint limit, you get to decide which foods to eat based on the SmartPoints value appointed to each meal. No foods are banned on the program, the only rule is not to go over your SmartPoints allowance. *Foods that are nutritious, healthy, and filling tend to have fewer SmartPoints, while high-fat, and high-carb meals tend to have larger SmartPoints value.*

This plan gives you the opportunity to choose healthy foods over the unhealthy ones. Some dieters even combine Weight loss with other diets such as the low-carb diet. It also means dieters won't have a hard time adopting this diet. You can follow the plan right this very second and it pretty much won't affect your day to day living.

The objective is to make better health decisions and lose weight in an unintimidating manner. It also heavily encourages including exercise and joining a support group. You are welcome to track your physical activity and exercise through activity trackers such as Fitbit. Here you will look at what exercise you are doing and how it will fit alongside your diet.

The third principle is joining a support group where you can meet like-minded people who share similar goals. You will also have a success coach watching over you who have been on the same journey as you. This is essential for the Weight loss program, and statistically, the more you attend the meetings, the higher your chance of weight loss success.

Weight loss: Foods You Can Eat

One reason why Weight loss Program is so popular is that there is no official restriction on what you can eat. The main objective of Weight loss is to keep track of your SmartPoints which helps control what you eat to lose weight.

Zero-point foods are foods that are low in saturated fat, sugar, carb, and calorie content. You should eat zero points foods as much as you can to help you lose weight, control your hunger, and stick with the Weight loss program. Here is the complete list of zero points foods which can help you make healthier food choices.

- Apples
- Unsweetened applesauce
- Apricots
- Arrowroots
- Artichoke hearts
- Artichokes
- Arugula
- Asparagus
- Bamboo shoots
- Banana
- Adzuki beans
- Black beans
- Green beans
- Chickpeas
- Great Northern beans
- Kidney beans
- Lima beans
- White beans

- Soybeans
- Navy beans
- Beets
- Berries
- Blackberries
- Blueberries
- Broccoli
- Brussel sprouts
- Green cabbage
- Red cabbage
- Bok choy
- Calamari
- Cantaloupe
- Carrots
- Cauliflower
- Caviar
- Celery
- Swiss chard
- Cherries
- Ground chicken breast
- Chicken breast or tenderloin
- Coleslaw mix
- Collards
- Corn
- White corn
- Cranberries
- Cucumber
- Daikon
- Dates
- Dragon fruit
- Egg substitutes
- Egg whites
- Eggplant
- Whole eggs
- Endive
- Fennel
- Figs
- Anchovies
- Sea Bass

- Carp
- Catfish
- Butterfish
- Cod
- Eel
- Haddock
- Halibut
- Herring
- Mackerel
- Monkfish
- Rainbow trout
- Rockfish
- Roe
- Salmon
- Sardines
- Seabass
- Striped mullet
- Swordfish
- Tuna
- Whitefish
- Tilapia
- Fruit cocktail
- Unsweetened fruit cup
- Fruit salad
- Unsweetened fruit
- Garlic
- Ginger root
- Grapefruit
- Grapes
- Honeydew melon
- Jackfruit
- Jerk chicken breast
- Kiwifruit
- Leeks
- Lemon
- Lemon zest
- Lentils
- Lettuce
- Lime

- Lime zest
- Mangoes
- Melon
- Brown mushrooms
- Button mushrooms
- Cremini mushrooms
- Italian mushrooms
- Portabella mushrooms
- Shiitake mushrooms
- Okra
- Onions
- Oranges
- Blood oranges
- Papayas
- Parsley
- Passionfruit
- Pears
- Peaches
- Peas
- Black-eyed peas
- Split peas
- Cayenne peppers
- Jalapeno peppers
- Poblano peppers
- Sweet bell peppers
- Pepperoncini
- Unsweetened pickles
- Pineapple
- Plumcots
- Plums
- Pomegranate seeds
- Pomegranate
- Pumpkin
- Pumpkin puree
- Radishes
- Radishes
- Raspberries
- Salsa verde
- Fat-free salsa

- Sauerkraut
- Scallions
- Seaweed
- Scallions
- Shallots
- Clams
- Crabs
- Crabmeat
- Crayfish
- Lobster
- Mussels
- Octopus
- Oysters
- Scallops
- Shrimp
- Squid
- Spinach
- Sprouts
- Summer squash
- Winter squash
- Zucchini
- Strawberries
- Tofu
- Tomatoes
- Tomato puree
- Tomato sauce
- Turkey
- Turnips
- Vegetable stick
- Mixed vegetables
- Water chestnuts
- Watermelon
- Greek yogurt
- Plain yogurt
- Soy yogurt

A Word of Caution on Zero Point Foods

Zero-point foods are the best thing about the Weight loss program but this may lead to slower weight loss. You should try to eat zero-point foods in moderation and only when you're hungry.

Do your best not to overeat and control your portion sizes even if it is zero-point foods. For example, while eggs are zero points, it isn't recommended to have an 8-egg omelet for breakfast.

Weight loss: Foods to Avoid

In the Weight loss, you should avoid foods with high SmartPoints value. Food that are high in refined carbs and fats and low protein tend to have a higher point value in the Weight loss program.

Such food items include cupcakes, cookies, ice cream, cheeseburgers, pasta, chili cheese fries, deep fried chicken, and cherry pies. Most foods served at fast food restaurants tend to have over 20 points! A triple whopper with cheese is 31 points!

So, what foods should you think twice on? Fast foods, junk foods, and sugary drinks are the absolute worst to eat if you want to feel satiated while cutting your caloric intake. This also includes many foods made with flour, gluten, or added sugar and most high-fat foods. These foods taste luxuriant but are loaded with fat and calories. Because of this, we eat them so fast that we eat too much before we feel satiated.

This doesn't mean you must cut all your favorite treats out of your diet entirely. Remember, you can eat anything on the Weight loss program, but only in moderation. Don't think you can eat a Bacon Cheeseburger Deluxe for lunch every day and expect to lose 2 pounds a week.

There are several useful strategies and advice that will help you get started on the Weight loss program. Below are top tips that will help you succeed in Weight loss:

Drink lots of water: Drinking water is essential for health, and it's going to help immeasurably in the Weight loss program. Drinking water also has many benefits including easier weight loss, clear skin, improved digestion, more energy, and increased mental clarity.

Learn portion control: Learning portion control is extremely important in Weight loss. You must be able to recognize ounces and cups when dining out or even cooking at home. If you can control portion and serving sizes, this can help ease the path to successful weight loss.

Don't overeat fruit: Fruits are zero SmartPoints food value because it is encouraged for dieters to eat them. They make good snacks and highly nutritious. So, don't be afraid to eat them. However, only eat fruit until you're satisfied, not full. It is recommended to eat only five servings of fruit per day.

Figure out your why: Motivation is crucial for weight loss. You will be more motivated to lose weight after you know why you want to lose weight in the first place. Some reasons include: having more energy, lowering your cholesterol, live longer, or look better. Find out why you committed to Weight loss program and remind yourself of it every day.

Don't guess SmartPoints: The most important thing to understand about SmartPoints is that you cannot guess SmartPoint values. The calculation of SmartPoints goes beyond calories. The calorie count you find on nutrition labels is based on the amount of energy in a food before it enters your body. After you consume it, your body processes it. As it processes the food, a portion of the food's calories is burned for body energy. Smart-Points are calculated based on the energy that is available after your body processed a food. This means you cannot just look at a food label and guess how much SmartPoints there is. You will over guess and throw the entire point system off balance.

Eat as many zero Points foods as you can: Take a look at the zero Points food list by Weight loss. There is plenty of tasty foods you can eat from and it's highly recommended to choose foods with zero points value whenever you can.

Don't cheat: If you want to eat something that is 9 points, and you only have 8 points left for the day, don't eat it believing it won't hurt you. It will really affect your body, diet, and mentality by adding that extra point. To find success in this program, you must be honest with yourself.

Share your journey: When you tell someone about your journey and progress, you are more likely to stay on track. You can participate in Weight loss meetings where you share your experience with other participants and leaders. You can even talk with someone, not on the diet, just someone who is supportive and makes you the most comfortable.

Plan your meals: By planning your meals ahead of time, it will help keep track of your SmartPoints throughout the day. If you're planning on dining out, figure out what you're going to order before you leave. If you're not a fan of meal prep, maybe you should start getting into the habit of it.

Track everything: Track your SmartPoints as you go. It's recommended that you carry a small notebook or have a tracking app on your phone. If you wait till before you sleep, you will probably forget some meals and snacks you had earlier today.

Don't forget exercise: Find ways to become more active and to move more in your life. When people lose weight through dieting, they tend to think that exercise is no longer necessary. They're wrong. You can lose weight quicker and become more fit if you include regular aerobic and cardio exercise in your life.

Expect progress, not perfection: Don't set yourself up for failure by seeking perfection. Don't set impossible goals. As you start the Weight loss program, you will go through days where you feel unmotivated and see no progress and you will go through days where you feel like you're on top of the world.

Be patient with yourself: While other diets may be too strict or just not working, the Weight loss program does work but it takes time to notice significant results. Remember, the Weight loss program is more of a lifestyle change than a diet. You won't find overnight success joining this program. You must be patient with yourself and not fight the change.

Eat high water content fruits and vegetables: If you can't drink a big jug of water, try eating high water content fruits and vegetables instead. Below you will find a list of high water content fruit and veggies.

Fruit and water content:

- Watermelon, 92% water content
- Strawberry, 92% water content
- Grapefruit, 91% water content
- Cantaloupe, 90% water content
- Peach, 88% water content
- Pineapple, 87% water content
- Cranberry, 87% water content
- Orange, 87% water content
- Raspberry, 87% water content
- Apricot, 86% water content
- Blueberry, 85% water content
- Plum, 85% water content
- Apple, 84% water content
- Pear, 84% water content
- Cherry, 81% water content
- Grape, 81% water content
- Banana, 74% water content

Veggies and water content:

- Cucumber, 96% water content
- Lettuce, 96% water content

- Zucchini, 95% water content
- Radish, 95% water content
- Celery, 95% water content
- Tomato, 94% water content
- Green cabbage, 93% water content
- Cauliflower, 92% water content
- Eggplant, 92% water content
- Red cabbage, 92% water content
- Pepper, 92% water content
- Spinach, 92% water content
- Broccoli, 91% water content
- Carrots, 87% water content
- Green pea, 79% water content
- Potato, 79% water content

Keep a Weight loss diary: Studies show that Weight loss participants who don't keep a food diary have a tougher time losing weight. It is recommended that you keep daily food records to successfully follow the Weight loss program and maintain steady weight loss.

I want you to find success with your health and your weight loss journey. In order to achieve this, you must follow the Weight loss program, but learn how to modify your entire way of thinking. The tips above will help you find ultimate success in your physical, mental, and financial health journey.

If you want to learn more dieting tips, look at WeightWatchers.com community message boards.

Chapter Two

OCTAVIA DIET

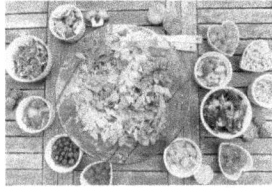

*T*he Octavia diet is a weight loss plan called "fueling" based on eating several meals a day. These mini-meals are brought and provided by the company which is meant to fill you up and help you shed pounds. A familiar sound? Octavia is an updated version that comes with a coach for those who are familiar with Medifast meal replacements. The convenience of replacing meal diets that take the guesswork out of the weight loss has long attracted consumers. The Octavia Diet is one prominent meal replacement plan. The Octavia Diet aims to aid people in losing weight by eating small amounts of calories throughout the day by combining "fueling" (shakes, bars, and other pre-packaged foods) with six small meals per-day philosophy.

By offering access to the health coach who will answer questions and provide encouragement, Octavia adds a social support component. As the name hasn't been around for a very long, the Octavia Diet might sound unfamiliar. You must have heard of the diet that was rebranded as Octavia in July 2017 under its previous name, Take Shape for Life. Take Shape for Life started as a subsidiary of the weight loss product company Medifast, which was found in 1980 by Dr. William Vitale, a medical doctor.

The intention of taking Shape for Life was to offer Medifast's products in an online format that was suited better to the digital age when it was introduced in 2002. Users who finish the program of Octavia are encouraged to become coaches, to sell the products of the company, and recruit new sales representatives.

How It Works

The Octavia Diet offers the users, like other meal replacement diets, its own array of branded products that take the place of several meals throughout the day. The "5 & 1" plan is the most common and it is intended for rapid weight loss. Users consume five of the "fuelings" of Octavia and one low-calorie "lean and green" homemade meal per day on this plan.

The other plans of Octavia, the "3 & 3" and "4 & 2 & 1", combine "real" meals with substitute. These plans are best for users who want to slowly lose their weight or maintain current weight.

Both "fueling", "lean and green" homemade meals are held with strict calorie ranges on all Octavia plans.

What to Eat

You can eat anywhere from two to five of the company's pre-made meal replacements ('fuelings') per day, depending on the Octavia diet plan you select. You will also prepare and eat one to three low-calorie meals of your own, which should mainly be lean protein and non-starchy vegetables.

Although no food is forbidden on a diet, many are strongly discouraged (such as sweets). There are also lots of foods, including healthy fats, that are highly recommended.

Compliant Foods

- Low-fat (on some plans) dairy, fresh fruit, and whole grains
- Fueling Octavia
- Healthy fats
- Greens and other vegetables that are not starchy
- Lean meats

Non-Compliant Foods

- Sugary drinks
- Alcohol
- Indulgent desserts
- Elevated-calorie additions

Compliant Foods

The majority of foods you eat from the diet plans of Octavia comes directly from the company, but you will also need to buy items to make your "lean and green" meal of the day.

Octavia "Fuelings"

The majority of foods you eat on the Octavia Diet will take the form of its "fuels" pre-packaged.

You can choose from over 60 soups, shakes, bars, pretzels, and other products (even brownies!) as meal replacements, according to Octavia's online guide.

The company shows that "each item has a nutrition profile that is almost identical," which means that they can be eaten interchangeably.

The Lean Meats

A five to seven-ounce portion of cooked lean protein must be included in the "lean and green" meals that you'll prepare. Using the following examples, Octavia distinguishes between lean, leaner, and leanest protein sources:

- Lean: Pork chops, lamb, or salmon
- Leaner: Breast of chicken or swordfish
- Leanest: Egg whites, shrimp, and cod

Non-Starchy and Green Vegetables

In your "lean and green" meal, Octavia's 5 & 1 program allows for two non-starchy vegetables alongside the protein.

The veggies are split into categories of lower, moderate, and higher carbohydrates, with the examples as follows:

- Lower Carb: Green Salads
- Moderate carb: Summer squash or cauliflower
- Higher Carb: Broccoli or peppers

Healthy Fats

A "lean and green" meal can be made with up to two servings of healthy fats, including olive or walnut oil, flaxseed, or avocado, in addition to lean protein and non-starchy vegetables.

Fresh Fruit, Low-Fat Dairy, and Whole Grains

"Once users have achieved their weight loss, they want to move on to a plan to maintain their weight through the meal replacements, lean protein, and non-starchy vegetables. Users can start reintroducing other food groups on Octavia's weight maintenance plans. Low-fat dairy, whole grains, and fresh fruit are all included in the weight maintenance programs of Octavia" 3 & 3 "and" 4 & 2 & 1.

Non-Compliant Foods

While the plans of Octavia do not prohibit specific foods, they do advise that you should avoid or restrict your intake of less healthy options that are unlikely to help your weight loss and do not provide valuable nutrition.

Indulgent Desserts

Not surprisingly, with sweets like cakes, cookies, or ice cream, Octavia discourages indulging your sugar cravings.

Moderate sweet treats such as fresh fruit or flavored yogurt can make their way back into your diet though after your initial weight loss phase

High-Calorie Additions

Butter, shortening, and high-fat salad dressings can add flavor, but they also contain large amounts of calories. You will be advised to keep additions to a minimum or replace lower-calorie versions on Octavia.

Sugary Drinks

Sweetened beverages such as juice, soda, or energy drinks provide calories without much satisfaction, so Octavia's plans are strongly discouraged.

Alcohol

The Octavia diet encourages alcohol restriction for users. A 5-ounce glass of red wine for 120 calories or 150 calories in a 12-ounce beer will quickly add up if you're trying to stay within a strict calorie range.

Resources and Products

Octavia offers resources in addition while providing your meal replacements that outline best practices for preparing your "lean and green" meals. Octavia maintains a Pinterest board of plan-compliant recipes if you need some fresh meal ideas.

The availability of a coach to cheer you throughout on your weight-loss trip is an additional resource that makes the Octavia program unique.

Modifications

The Octavia diet relies on meal replacement products and the meals that are prepared strictly to control calories, so there is not much room for modification. Fatigue, brain fog, headaches, or menstrual changes can be caused by extreme calorie restriction. As such, long-term use of the 5 & 1 option should not be used.

However, typically, the 3 & 3 and 4 & 2 & 1 plans provide between 1100 to 2500 calories per day and can be suitable for a longer period of use.

Pros

- Offers social aid
- Takes out the guesswork on what to eat
- Achieves rapid weight reduction
- Packaged goods provide convenience

Cons

- Mealtimes may become dull or it feels isolated.
- Limiting calories can leave you hungry or tired.
- Includes a great deal of processed food
- Losing weight may be unsustainable.
- High monthly costs

Pros

If you need a diet plan that is clear and easy to follow, which will help you to quickly lose weight, and offers built-in social support, Octavia's program might fit well for you.

Offer Convenience from packaged products

The shakes, soups, and all other meal replacement products from Octavia are delivered directly to your door, a level of convenience that is not provided by many other diets.

Although you will have to shop for your ingredients for "lean and green" meals, the home delivery options for Octavia's "fuelings" saves energy and time. Once the products have arrived, they're very easy to prepare and make an excellent grab and go meals.

Achieves quick weight loss

In order to maintain their weight loss, most healthy people need about 1600 to 3000 calories per day. Restricting that figure to as low as 800 essentially guarantees most people's weight loss.

The 5 & 1 plan of Octavia is intended for rapid weight loss, making it a solid option for someone with a medical reason to quickly lose pounds.

Removes Guesswork

Some people discover that the most difficult part of dieting is the mental effort needed to figure out what to eat every day or even in every meal.

Octavia alleviates the tension and stress of meal planning and "decision fatigue" by offering "fueling", "lean and green" meal guidelines to users with the clear cut approved foods.

Offers Social Support

With any weight loss plan, social support is a vital component of success. The coaching program and group calls from Octavia provide built-in encouragement and support users.

Cons

Octavia's plan also has some potential downsides, particularly if you are worried about cost, flexibility, and variety.

Monthly High Cost

The expense of Octavia can be a deterrent to prospective users. For 119 servings, the 5 & 1 plan ranges in price from $350 to $425.

As you consider the cost of the program, don't forget to take into your account that the food you will need to buy to prepare your "lean and green" meals.

Includes Processed Food

Although the 'fuelings' of Octavia are engineered with interchangeable nutrients, they are still undeniably processed foods, which may be a turn-off for some users.

Nutrition research has shown that eating a lot of processed food can have harmful effects on one's health, so there may be a disadvantage to this aspect of the diet plan.

May not be sustainable weight loss.

One challenge that anyone on a diet is familiar is with how to determine and maintain weight loss once the program is completed.

For Octavia's program, the same goes. When users return to eat regular meals instead of meal replacements from the plan, they may find that they quickly regain the weight that they have lost.

Calorie Restriction Effects

Although Octavia's diet plan emphasizes to frequently eat throughout the day, only 110 calories are provided by each of its "fuels." "Lean and green" meals are low in calories as well.

If you generally eat fewer calories, you may find that the plan leaves you hungry and unsatisfied. You can also feel tired and even irritable more easily.

Isolation and boredom at mealtimes

The social aspects of cooking and eating food can interfere with Octavia's dependence on meal replacements.

At a family mealtime or when you are dining out with friends, users may find it awkward or disappointing to have a shake or a bar.

How does it compare

The Octavia Diet can be more efficient than other plans for rapid weight loss simply because of how few calories its fuels that "lean and green" meals provide.

In the US, Octavia was ranked by News and World Report as the second-best rapid weight loss diet.

Octavia requires less "mental gymnastics" than competitors such as Weight loss (for which you need to learn a point system) or keto (for which you need to monitor and evaluate macronutrients closely).

The coaching component of Octavia is comparable to Weight loss and Jenny Craig, both of which encourage participants to opt in to get social support for meetings. Compared to the array of fresh and whole foods you can eat more on self-guided plans like Atkins, the highly processed nature of most foods you will eat on the Octavia diet can be a downside.

Recommendations from USDA

In several areas, the Octavia Diet deviates from the health and nutrition guidelines which are encouraged by the Department of Agriculture of the United States (USDA).

Although the 5 & 1 plan by Octavia is intended for weight loss, the calorie count of 800 to 1000 per day is an extreme reduction from the USDA's recommendation.

In terms of macronutrients, specifically, carbohydrates, one area where Octavia deviates from USDA recommendations.

Reportedly, Octavia's plans provide 80 to 100 grams of carbohydrates per day. About 30 percent of the daily calories in the diet come from carbs, whereas a diet that is 45 to 65 percent carbohydrates is recommended by the USDA Dietary Guidelines.

The USDA also stresses that grains and dairy products that are not represented in the 5 & 1 plan of Octavia are included in a healthy eating plan.

How successful is the Octavia Diet?

"Some may appeal for this program because it does not require carbs or calories to be tracked," says by the registered dietician Summer Yule. "With this program, participants may also see quick weight loss because the dietary component is so low in calories (in some cases, 800 to 1,000 calories per day). They also receive some coaching behavioral support that can be helpful in weight loss. Previous research has given that ongoing coaching can help individuals to lose weight both in the short and long term.

One 16-week study (that was founded by Medifast, the company behind Octavia) found that compared to the control group, participants with the excess weight or obesity on the 5&1 Plan of Octavia had significantly lower weight, fat levels, and waist circumference. The same research also found that those on the 5&1 diet who completed at least 75% of the coaching sessions have lost more than twice the weight of those participating in fewer sessions.

What do you eat on Octavia?

Its 'fuelings,' which include bars, shakes, cookies, cereal, and some savory options, such as soup and mashed potatoes, comprise at least half of any Octavia diet. These processed foods often list the first ingredient as soy protein or whey protein.

The rest of the diet you purchase and prepare on your own is filled with lean and green meals. These include:

- 5-7 ounces of lean protein cooked, such as fish, chicken, egg whites, turkey, or soya
- Three servings of lettuce, greens, celery, or cucumbers of non-starchy vegetables
- Up to 2 servings of healthy fats such as olive oil, avocado, or olives

CHAPTER TWO: BENEFITS OF OCTAVIA DIET

While you lose weight on this diet, you may also feel hungry. "The downside of this is that an extreme, and usually unhealthy, calorie reduction is required," Derocha says. If you're looking to lose weight, that may sound fine, but she warns that you may miss vitamins, minerals, fiber, and antioxidants. "With the prepackaged meals and the extreme reduction in calories, these are imbalanced or lost."

What are the long and short-term effects of the Octavia Diet?

In the short term, because of the calorie limit, you might lose weight quickly, says Derocha. "However, users may also experience side effects of malnutrition, such as hair loss, impaired appearance of the skin, constipation, dehydration, headaches, and fatigue for the same reason. There is a risk of immune deficiency that leads to more frequent illnesses, she says.

Can Constipation be Caused by the Octavia Diet?

The good news regarding the diet of Octavia is that the products of Octavia, lean and Green meals encourage the consumption of vegetables containing digestion-friendly fiber. But Derocha points out that a few people with gastrointestinal discomfort may be left with the addition of whey and soy in prepackaged products. It is unlikely that the Octavia diet will help you to maintain weight loss in the long term. "On this type of diet, the probability of regaining the weight is greater than if you learn portion control and healthy eating lifestyle habits on your own."

Is Octavia a Ketogenic Diet?

No, like the ketogenic diet, the Octavia diet is not an extremely low carbohydrate diet. You eat a lot of fat, a small amount of protein, and very few carbs on a keto diet. This meal plan means eating no fruit, no cereals such as bread, rice, and plenty of high-fat foods such as avocado, meat, and olive oil.

Reviews of Octavia Diet: Where Do Registered Dietitians Stand?

The Octavia diet, Young says, is not a perpetual diet and it has some deeper flaws. A single protein and green meal are healthy, and the overall diet could be used to give someone a quick jump-start. But it's over-processed, and the focus on prepackaged food choices never teaches anyone how to eat,' she says. Ultimately, Young says, "Eating doesn't have to be like this."

The Octavia diet is a set of three programs, two of which focus on weight loss and one that is best for maintaining weight. In order to encourage weight loss, the plans are higher in protein and lower in carbo-hydrates and calories. Each plan requires to eat at least half of your food in the form of Octavia prepackaged food. Since the plan calls for carbs, protein, and fat to be eaten, it is also a fairly balanced plan for food groups.

As far as weight loss goes, experts say that while Octavia can help because it's lower in calories, for the better, it's unlikely to permanently alter your eating habits. You're likely to regain the weight once you stop your diet.

In addition, experts like Derocha warn that there may not be enough calories in this model to meet the needs of your body.

Does the Octavia Diet have any health hazards?

Studies have not shown major Octavia problems. Side effects for those are at risk, constipation, and (for women) menstrual changes could include leg cramps, dizziness or fatigue, headaches, loose skin, hair loss, rashes, gas, diarrhea, bad breath, gallstones, or gallbladder disease.

The apparent lack of noteworthy risks does not mean that Octavia is safe for all. There should be no programs for pregnant women and those who are younger than 13 years of age, while teenagers, nursing mothers, people with gout, and others should stick to those programs aimed at them (after clearing up with their doctors, of course). The 5&1 program should be avoided by older, sedentary adults and individuals who exercise for more than 45 minutes a day. Unless their health care providers have approved them as recovered and stabilized, individuals with serious diseases such as cancer, liver disease, kidney disease, or an eating disorder should not follow any plan.

Before starting any of the programs, the company advises, if you are on any medications, particularly warfarin, lithium, diabetes medication, or high blood pressure medications, you should talk to your doctor first.

Is the Octavia Diet a healthy diet for the heart?

Octavia may be healthy for your heart, but not more than many other diets. Octavia claims that its fuels are low in fat and cholesterol, and it may contain sufficient high-quality soy protein to meet the Heart Health claim of the Food and Drug Administration.

Octavia represents the coaching community and the Medifast lifestyle brand that was launched in 2017. Previous studies have been conducted by using products from Medifast, not new products from Octavia. While the products from Octavia represent a new line, Medifast has advised the U.S. News that they have an identical profile of macronutrients and are interchangeable with Medifast products. Therefore, when evaluating this diet, we believe that these studies are relevant.

Participants decreased their blood pressure significantly. In the 2017 Medifast-sponsored study in the journal Nutrition and Diabetes.

A 2015 study carried out by Medifast and it was found that overweight and obese participants significantly improved their blood pressure following the 4&2&1 plan.

Researchers reported declines in the blood pressure, pulse rate, and blood levels of C-reactive protein, a marker of inflammation that can predict heart disease risk, in the Medifast and control groups at week 40, in the 2010 Nutrition Journal study described in the weight-loss section. The study also reported on the size of the waist and the amount of abdominal fat that are believed to be indicators of the risk of heart diseases. Medifast dieters lost an average of about 4 inches around the waist at week 40, with the control group losing about 1 1/2 inches. For both groups, the abdominal' fat rate' also decreased, but the Medifast group performed slightly better. For the Medifast group, total cholesterol was not significantly lower at week 40, but for the control group, it had dropped significantly. At 40 weeks, neither group showed improved levels of triglycerides, a fatty substance that has been excessively associated with heart disease.

The Medifast dieters were significantly higher in good HDL cholesterol and lower systolic blood pressure after 86 weeks in the Diabetes Educator study, but no change was significant compared to the control group.

Can diabetes be prevented or controlled by the Octavia Diet?

Octavia may be able to prevent or control diabetes, but research does not demonstrate an advantage over other diets.

Prevention: One of the biggest risk factors for Type 2 diabetes is being overweight. If Octavia helps you to lose weight and keep it off, in your favor, you can help to tilt the odds.

The preliminary findings of the study on waist circumference and abdominal fat from the Nutrition Journal, cited in the cardiovascular section, it was suggested that Medifast dieters may be able to reduce two risk factors associated with diabetes. In the journal Nutrition and Diabetes, the 2017 Medifast-sponsored study, and it was found that both individuals with and without type 2 diabetes decreased their body fat, blood pressure, pulse, and waist circumference significantly.

Control: Octavia offers specific diabetic plans; the number of calories, carbohydrates, and lean and green meals they provide is similar or slightly different from the typical adult plan. The Diabetes Educator study described in the weight loss section which has shown favorable short-term changes in the blood while fasting, glucose, and insulin levels of Medifast dieters at 34 weeks, but the changes had all but disappeared at 86 weeks.

Does the Octavia Diet allow for preferences and restrictions?

For more information, most dieters will find an Octavia program that fits their needs to choose your preference.

Recommended supplement? You should not need an Octavia supplement, but if you are already taking one per by the recommendation of a health care provider, check with the provider to see if your regimen should continue or adjust.

Vegetarian: On Octavia, staying or going vegetarian is doable if you are willing to accept a limited menu of products from Octavia. Octavia offers resources to make your lean and green meals vegetarian, but since you are asked to avoid good sources of plant-based proteins such as peas, beans, and lentils as they are too high in carbohydrates, it won't necessarily be easy.

Vegan: There is no plan to eat Octavia vegan, and it is not recommended. Octavia Fuelings has a per-mix vitamin D derived from lanolin (sheep's wool).

Gluten-Free: Octavia can be gluten-free. Some fuels, including selected shakes, soups, bars, and pudding that have been certified as gluten-free.

Low-Salt: All plans should be low-sodium friendly, with some extra attention to be paid for the preparation of lean & green foods.

Kosher: Some kosher pareve and kosher milk options are offered by Octavia.

Halal: Octavia Fuelings are not halal, but the kosher options may work for dieters.

Is there a nutritious Octavia Diet?

Experts concluded that it does not perfectly align with the federal government's healthy eating guidelines because it provides too much protein and few carbs too. At 800 to 1,000 calories a day, it also dips low for many dieters. That's less than half the amount recommended for men from 21 to 40 in the federal guidelines and almost that much less for women in that age group. The experts have found it "moderately" secure.

In addition to suggestions from the federal government in 2015. Dietary Guidelines for Americans, here is a breakdown of the nutritional content of a day of meals on the Optimal Weight 5&1 Plan.

Is the diet for Octavia healthy?

What has considered a high-protein diet is the Octavia diet, with a protein making up to 10-35 percent of your daily calories. The processed powdered type, however, can lead to some less pleasant implications.

In a smoothie, London says, "The protein isolate plus additives can make you feel bloated and have some other unwanted GI side effects, making you better off with unsweetened Greek yogurt for protein."

Plus, for safety and efficacy, the FDA does not regulate dietary supplements such as shakes and powders the same way it does for the food. "Powders and blends of protein may have undesirable ingredients, or may interact with a drug you may be taking," London adds, "making it extra important to make sure your doctor knows that you are trying the plan."

How is Octavia supposed to help you lose weight?

To promote weight loss, Octavia relies on intensively restricting calo-ries. Most "fuels" contain about 100-110 calories each, which means you can consume about 1,000 calories per day on this diet.

The U.S. due to the dramatic approach of Octavia, News and World Report ranked second for the Best Fast Weight-Loss Diets list, but # 32 in it is the Best Healthy Eating Diets list. "It seems impossible not to reduce at least a few pounds in the short term; you're eating half of the calories most adults eat," it said. "The outlook for the long term is less promising."

"Eating meals and snacks includes loads of produce, 100 percent whole grains, nuts, seeds, legumes, and pulses, low-fat dairy products, eggs, poul-try, seafood, and lean beef, plus some indulgences, it is the best way to sustainably lose weight for the long haul."

How much water am I supposed to drink? What about other drinks?

Each day, we recommend you to drink 64 ounces of water. Before changing the amount of water you drink, talk to your healthcare provider, as it can affect certain health conditions and medications.

On what counts towards hydration, there are many different recom-mendations and points of view. That's because your body gets water from the foods you eat and the drinks you consume, in addition to your daily drinking water, all of which contribute to your overall hydration status. As water plays a major role in supporting our health, we recommend drinking 64 ounces of water every day. Water helps to remove waste from the body and clean all of our organs and systems function properly by being well-hydrated. Water is a critical component of the body, making up between 55 and 60% of our body weight, according to Dr. A's Habits of Health. Since our bodies are unable to store water, we often need to replenish it, which is why drinking 64 ounces of water each day is one of the key health habits.

So, while other calorie and carbohydrate-free drinks, such as unsweet-ened tea and coffee, may be available on the Octavia program and techni-cally contribute to your overall hydration, we still recommend that you should drink 64 ounces of water each day. Hydration needs, vary from person to person, so we encourage you to listen to your body for addi-tional guidance and talk to your healthcare provider.

Purpose Hydration

One healthy habit really leads to another at Octavia. We succeed in everything we do by incorporating healthy habits. We have products that make it easier, and we have coaches who inspire and teaches you. The key to successful habit creation is repetition. And what makes repetition possible is the purpose.

Every commodity has two purposes. With your life at once. First purpose: to tell you when and why to hydrate yourself. The second purpose: to remain hydrated all day long.

We should make healthy hydration our second nature, just like healthy eating. When You get to the place you need to go with proven nutrition and purposeful hydration. Our Octavia trainers make sure you never go alone with it.

On the Octavia program, what condiments and healthy fats can I have?

Recommendations on Condiment

To add flavor and zest to your meals, use condiments; just remember that they contribute to your overall intake of carbohydrates. For optimal outcomes, we recommend reading food labels for carbohydrate information and controlling condiment portions. A serving of condiments should not contain more than 1 gram per serving of carbohydrates. On all plans, you can have three condiment servings per lean and green meal daily.

Recommendations on Healthy Fat

Monounsaturated and polyunsaturated fats are considered more beneficial to your health than saturated fats, such as olive oil, olives, nuts,seeds, and avocado. From those two categories, we recommend you to choose most of your healthy fat servings. There should be around 5 grams of fat and less than 5 grams of carbohydrate in a healthy fat serving. Depending on the lean protein choices, you will have 0-2 servings of healthy fats per lean and green meal.

While on the Octavia Program, can I dine out?

Meals for special occasions are simple to handle than you might think! Simply rearrange your fueling routine (if necessary) at your breakfast meeting, family brunch, awards banquet, family dinner at a restaurant, or virtually on any special occasion involving food, you can enjoy your lean and green food!

You should have your typical lean and green meal when dining out, consisting of 5 to 7 ounces of cooked lean protein, three servings of non-starchy vegetables, and depending on your lean choices, 0-2 servings of healthy fats. Request that your meat should be prepared/served without sauces and added fats; you can switch to lower carbohydrate choices (such as steamed broccoli or green beans) for starchy vegetable options (such as potatoes). Ask your server to skip the chips breadbasket or a bowl and get your salad dressing on your side at all the times.

At popular fast food and sit-down restaurants, our Dining Out Guide has specific lean and green meal menu recommendations as well as additional tips on how to make healthy choices when you are dining out.

It may increase your daily calorie intake if you can't avoid eating something that isn't part of the lean and green meal, but you can get back on your Octavia plan, starting with your next meal. Even when you think you may have over-eaten, it is still best not to skip meals. As soon as you are able to start, resume your strategy.

As an alternative, when you dine out and ask the waiter for hot or cold water (depending on what you are eating) to mix with your Fueling, you can bring along your own a Fueling and then just make your Fueling ready and eat it with everyone else!

While on the Octavia program, should I exercise?

Exercise is a significant aspect of weight loss, metabolic process improvement, and weight loss maintenance. Exercise also offers a lot of health benefits, such as improve control of blood sugar, improve flexibility and balance, control of blood pressure, strength, and endurance, and helps you to reduce stress.

If you are not exercising regularly when starting the Octavia program, we recommend that you wait two to three weeks before starting the exercise program (and check with your healthcare provider). Start an exercise program calmly and gradually increase the time spent on an activity as your body allows (and the intensity of the activity). Choose an activity you can regularly enjoy. Most of our customers find that walking is the easiest activity they can integrate into their everyday life.

For an individual who has an exercise program in place before starting our program, we recommend cutting your exercise program intensity and duration in half for the first few weeks to allow the body to adjust to its new calorie level.

As your body adapts to this lower-calorie level, the time and intensity of your exercise plan can be increased. We recommend 30 minutes of moderate exercise for the entire time you are on the Optimal Weight 5 & 1 Plan while limiting exercise to 45 minutes of light to moderate physical activity each day.

Listen to your body system and do what it only allows. If you feel lightheaded or faint stop your workout and take a rest before you resume.

What if I have a night shift at work or a long day?

If you are working on a night shift or have long days, you can rearrange your fueling schedule to suit your schedule. The most important thing in Octavia that in a 24-hour period you consume all of your Octavia Fuelings and the complete lean and green meal. Try to eat as much as possible after every 2 to 3 hours whenever you are awake. You can split the lean and green food into two smaller meals if you want you can eat a total of 7 meals instead of 6. If required, you may also incorporate an optional snack. For further guidance and support, be sure to speak with your Octavia coach.

What happens if I'm a vegetarian?

There are a lot of Octavia Fuelings to fit in your lifestyle, whether you adopt a vegetarian diet for health, ecological, religious, or ethical reasons. 24 + vitamins and minerals, including iron, vitamin B12, zinc, calcium, vitamin D, and riboflavin, are fortified and contain 11-15 grams of high-quality protein.

As outlined on the Meatless Options List on the Vegetarian Information Sheet, you can make your lean and green meal(s) vegetarian by using meatless options. If you are part of the Optimal Weight 5 & 1 Plan, until you reach your goal of weight loss, you should avoid legumes (peas, beans, lentils, etc.) as these foods are too high in carbohydrates to keep you in a state of fat burning. While on the Optimal Health 3 & 3 Plan, these foods can be reintroduced.

What if I miss the Fueling?

It is very vital that you get all your Fuelings every day and the full portions of your lean and green meals. You may need to space the rest of your meals close together if you miss a meal to ensure that you get the rest of your meals before the end of the day.

It won't help to increase your weight loss by skipping meals; it may actually have the opposite effect! If you have to decide between "skipping" a meal or "doubling up" make sure that you get within a 24-hour period all of your Fuelings and lean and green meals, it is better to double up (eat two Fuelings at the same time) than to miss one of the Fuelings' nutrition.

What is the best starting day?

Depending on what fits best for you, you can begin on any day. For your success, the first few days are critical, so pick a start date that makes sense for your schedule. You may want to look for a time when you do not expect any family, job-related, or other events of a social type that may present additional barriers or temptations. Let your Octavia coach know which day you are planning to start so, that they can give you guidance and support.

Chapter Three

CHRONIC KIDNEY DISEASE

*C*hronic Kidney Disease (CKD) cannot be cured as damages to parts of our kidneys are usually irreversible. However, the good news is that you can slow down the progression of its critical stages by embracing a new lifestyle and changing your way of eating. The kind of foods we eat indubitably has a great effect on the health of our body organs, including the kidneys. As a chronic kidney disease patient, the best thing to do is to switch to a kidney-friendly diet. This kind of diet is popularly known as the Renal Diet.

A proper Renal Diet is a non-medicinal solution to kidney problems. It is both preventive and restrictive to help treat kidney disease by controlling the consumption of kidney-damaging elements like sodium, potassium, and phosphorous. While these minerals are important for maintaining blood pressure, hydration, nerve impulses, and hormone regulation, too much can burden the kidneys and eventually damage kidney cells called nephrons. The Renal Diet works to protect our kidneys.

Firstly, this specific diet calls for lower sodium consumption by restricting salts and products high in salt. It also proposes lower potassium consumption by restricting high-potassium salt substitutes and canned items. Similarly, it also limits phosphorus consumption in excessive amounts. The recipes shared in this book are created with these limits in mind.

Secondly, the diet prohibits all food that could indirectly affect kidney health related to high blood pressure, edema, heart problems, diabetes, etc. High amounts of protein can contribute to kidney damage once they are digested since they produce toxic substances, therefore the Renal Diet recommends reducing protein consumption as much as possible.

Moreover, fruits, vegetables, juices, and water play an important role in the Renal Diet. Drinking more fluids creates an environment inside the kidneys that provide instant relief to damaged or strained kidney cells. Exercise and physical activity also play their part in making this diet effective as they help improve your metabolism and break down the food you eat more.

Although CKD cannot be cured, the Renal Diet can help patients retain their kidney functions and delay kidney failure for years. The major effect of the Renal Diet on our kidneys is that it reduces the workload of the kidney, thereby making them function better and longer.

RENAL DIET BENEFITS

Dietary control, including protein, phosphorus, and sodium limitation, when combined with the veggie lover nature of the renal eating regimen and keto acid supplementation, can conceivably apply a cardiovascular defensive impact in perpetual renal disappointment patients by following up on both conventional and nontraditional cardiovascular hazard factors.

Circulatory strain control might be supported by the decrease of sodium consumption and the vegan idea of the eating routine, which is significant for bringing down serum cholesterol and improving the plasma lipid profile. The low protein and phosphorus admission have a significant job for decreasing proteinuria and forestalling and switching hyperphosphatemia and auxiliary hyperparathyroidism, which are real reasons for the vascular calcifications, cardiovascular harm, and mortality danger of uremic patients.

The decrease of nitrogenous waste items and bringing down serum PTH levels may likewise help enhance insulin affectability and metabolic control in diabetic patients, just as increment the responsiveness to erythropoietin treatment, which accordingly permits more noteworthy control of iron deficiency. Likewise, protein-limited eating regimens may have calming and antioxidant properties.

Accordingly, setting aside the still begging to be proven bad consequences for the movement of renal ailment and the more conceded impacts on uremic signs and side effects, it is conceivable that an appropriate healthful treatment right off the bat throughout renal sickness might be helpful additions to diminish the cardiovascular hazard in the renal patient. Be that as it may, definitive information can't yet be drawn because quality investigations are deficient in this field, future examinations ought to be intended to evaluate the impact of renal eating regimens on hard results, as cardiovascular occasions or mortality.

Basic principles

The general principles of diet treatment for chronic kidney patients are as follows:

- Limit protein intake to 0.8 gm/kg per kilogram per day for non-dialysis patients. Patients on dialysis need a greater amount of protein to compensate for the possible loss of proteins during the procedure. (1.0 to 1.2 gm/kg daily according to body weight)
- Taking enough carbohydrates to provide energy.
- Taking normal amounts of oil. Reduction of butter, pure fat, and oil intake.
- Restriction of fluid and water intake in case of swelling (edema).
- Dietary intake of sodium, potassium, and phosphorus limitation.
- Taking adequate amounts of vitamins and trace elements. A high-fiber diet is recommended.

The details of the selection and modification of the diet for chronic kidney patients are as follows:

High-Calorie Intake

In addition to daily activities, the body needs calories to maintain heat, growth, and adequate body weight. Calories are taken with carbohydrates and fats. According to body weight, the daily normal calorie intake of patients suffering from chronic kidney disease is 35-40 kcal/kg. If caloric intake is insufficient, the body uses proteins to provide calories. Such protein distribution may cause harmful effects, such as improper nutrition and increased production of waste materials. Therefore, it is very important to provide sufficient calories to CKD patients. It is important to calculate the patient's daily calorie requirement based on the ideal body weight, not the current weight.

Carbohydrates

Carbohydrates are the primary source of calories required for the body.

Carbohydrates, wheat, cereals, rice, potatoes, fruits and vegetables, sugar, honey, cookies, pastry, confectionery, and beverages. Diabetes and obesity patients should limit the number of carbohydrates. It is best to use complex carbohydrates that can be obtained from whole grains such as whole wheat or raw rice that can provide fiber. They should constitute a large part of the number of carbohydrates in the diet. The proportion of all other sugar-containing substances should not exceed 20% of the total carbohydrate intake, particularly in diabetic patients. If chocolate, hazelnut, or banana desserts are consumed in a limited amount, non-diabetic patients may be replaced with calories, fruit, pies, pastry, cookies, and protein.

Oils

Fats are an important source of calories for the body and provide twice as many calories as carbohydrates and proteins. Chronic kidney patients should limit the intake of saturated fat and cholesterol that may cause heart disease. In unsaturated fat, it is necessary to pay attention to the proportion of monounsaturated fat and polyunsaturated fat. Excessive uptake of omega-6 polyunsaturated fatty acids (CFAs) and a relatively high omega-6 / omega-3 ratio are detrimental, while the low omega-6 / omega-3 ratio has beneficial effects. The use of vegetable oils instead of uniform oils will achieve this goal. Trans fat-containing substances such as potato chips, sweet buns, instant cookies, and pastries are extremely dangerous and should be avoided.

Restriction of Protein Intake

Protein is essential for the restoration and maintenance of body tissues. It also helps to heal wounds and fight infection. In patients with chronic renal failure who do not undergo dialysis, protein limitation is recommended to reduce the rate of decrease in renal function and postpone the need for dialysis and renal transplantation. (<0.8 gm/kg daily according to body weight). However, excessive protein restriction should also be avoided due to the risk of malnutrition.

Anorexia is a common condition in patients with chronic kidney disease. Strict protein restriction, poor diet, weight loss, fatigue, loss of body resistance, and loss of appetite increase the risk of death. High protein proteins such as animal protein (meat, poultry, and fish), eggs, and tofu are preferred. Chronic kidney patients should avoid high protein diets (e.g., the Atkins diet). Similarly, protein supplements or medications such as creatinine used for muscle development should be avoided unless recommended by a physician or dietician. However, as the patient begins dialysis, daily protein intake should be increased by 1.0 to 1.2 gm/kg body weight to recover the proteins lost during the procedure.

Fluid intake

- Why should chronic kidney patients take precautions about fluid intake?

The kidneys play an important role in maintaining the correct amount of water in the body by removing excess liquid as urea. In patients with chronic kidney disease, the urea volume usually decreases as the kidney functions deteriorate. Reduction of urea excretion from the body causes fluid retention in the body, resulting in facial swelling, swelling of legs and hands, and high blood pressure. Accumulation of fluid in the lungs (called pulmonary obstruction or edema) causes shortness of breath and difficulty breathing. This can be life-threatening if not checked.

- What precautions should chronic kidney patients take to control fluid intake?

To prevent overloading or loss of fluid, the amount of fluid taken on a physician's advice should be recorded and monitored. The amount of water to be taken for each chronic kidney patient may vary, and this rate is calculated according to the urea excretion and fluid status of each patient.

- What is the recommended amount of fluid for patients with chronic kidney disease?

Unlimited edema and water intake can be done in patients who do not have edema and can throw enough urea from the body. It is a common misconception that patients with kidney disease should take large amounts of water and fluids to protect their kidneys. The recommended amount of fluid depends on the patient's clinical condition and renal function.

Patients with edema who cannot appoint sufficient urea from the body should limit fluid intake. To reduce swelling, fluid intake within 24 hours should be less than the amount of urine produced by the daily body.

In patients with edema, the amount of fluid that should be taken daily should be 500 ml more than the other day's urine volume to prevent fluid overload or fluid loss. This additional 500 ml of liquid will approximately compensate for the fluids lost by perspiration and exhalation.

- Why should chronic kidney patients keep a record of their daily weight?

Patients need to record their weight daily to detect fluid increase or loss or to monitor fluid volume in their bodies. Bodyweight will remain constant if the instructions for fluid intake are strictly followed. Sudden weight gain indicates excessive fluid overload due to increased fluid intake in the body. Weight gain is a warning that the patient should make more rigorous fluid restriction. Weight loss is usually caused by fluid restriction and the use of diuretics.

Useful Tips for Restricting Fluid Intake

1. Reduce salty, spicy, or fried foods in your diet because these foods can increase your thirst and cause more fluid consumption.
2. Only for water when you are thirsty. Do not drink as a habit or because everyone drinks.
3. When thirsty, consume only a small amount of water or try ice — sure, taking a little ice cube. Ice stays in the mouth longer than water to give a more satisfying result than the same amount of water. Remember to calculate the amount of liquid consumed. To calculate simply, freeze the amount of water allocated for drinking in the ice block.
4. To prevent dry mouth, gargle with water, but do not swallow the water. Dry mouth can also be reduced by chewing gum, sucking hard candies, lemon slices, or mint candies, and using a small amount of water to moisturize your mouth.
5. Always use small cups or glasses to limit fluid intake. Instead of consuming extra water for medication use, take your medicines while drinking water after meals.
6. The patient should engage himself in a job. Patients who are not engaged in a job often desire to drink water.
7. High blood sugar in diabetic patients can increase the level of thirst. To reduce thirst, it is essential to keep blood sugar under tight control.

8. Since the person's thirst increases in hot weather, measures to be in cooler environments may be preferred and recommended.

WHAT YOU NEED TO MONITOR WITH RENAL DIET

Should you choose to accept it, your mission is to ensure that you minimize waste buildup in your kidneys. To do that, you need to watch what you eat, carefully preparing or arranging your meals so that you receive the required nutrition, minus all the unnecessary components.

This is where a Renal Diet becomes an essential component of your life.

Before delving deeper into the diet itself, let us look at some of the important substances that people with CKD need to manage.

Sodium

Suppose you have been enjoying your pasta, nachos, pizzas, juicy steaks, lip-smacking burgers, or practically any of your favorite savory food items. In that case, the chances are that you have been consuming sodium. Why? Well, this mineral is commonly found in salt. Whether you use table salt or sea salt, you are going to find sodium in them.

If you have heard people claim that sodium is harmful to your body, let me tell you that it is not entirely true. We need sodium in our bodies. The mineral helps our body maintain a balance in the levels of water within and around our cells. At the same time, it also maintains your blood pressure levels.

Surprised? You might have thought that sodium makes things worse, but there is a medical condition called hyponatremia, or "low blood sodium." When sodium levels drop to a low enough level, then you experience all the symptoms below:

- Weakness
- Nausea
- Vomiting
- Fatigue or low energy
- Headache
- Irritability
- Muscle cramps or spasms
- Confusion

In conclusion, sodium is essential for your body. However, when you are on a Renal Diet, you control the amount of salt that you add to your food. Since the kidneys are rather sensitive at this point, there is no need to exacerbate their condition by adding more sodium.

This might prove difficult for people since they are used to having salt as a flavoring ingredient in their foods. But that is why we will use recipes full of flavors that you will enjoy (more on that when we get started on the recipes).

Potassium

Potassium is one of those minerals that people might not think about too much compared to calcium or sodium, but it nonetheless serves an important role in our body.

Apart from regulating fluids in the body, it also aids in passing messages between the body and brain. Like sodium, potassium is classified as an electrolyte, a term used to refer to a family of minerals that react in water. When potassium is dissolved in water, it produces positively charged ions. Using these ions, potassium can conduct electricity, which allows it to carry out some incredibly important functions. Take, for example, the messages that are communicated between the brain and the body. These messages are sent back and forth in the form of impulses. However, one must wonder, what exactly creates those impulses? It's not as if our body has an inbuilt electrical generator.

The answer lies in the ions. We have already established that sodium and potassium are both electrolytes and produce ions. The impulses are created when sodium ions move into the cells, and potassium ions move out of the cell. This movement changes the voltage of the cell, producing impulses. The way the impulses are created is like Morse code but takes place much faster (it has to for your body to react, manage processes, or perform tasks). When the level of potassium falls, the body's ability to generate nerve impulses gets affected.

Wait a minute. So, potassium is good. Does that mean I am asking you to let your body give up on normal nerve impulses to keep your kidneys safe? Is that the only choice? That's a tough choice to make!

Relax. What we are going to do is avoid having too much potassium.

When the kidneys are not functioning properly, then their potassium buildup could cause problems to the heart. More specifically, they could change the heartbeats' rhythm, leading to a potential heart attack. You mustn't worry though; this does not happen with just a mild increase in potassium. There must be a significant increase to cause such a devastating result.

Nevertheless, we are going to avoid even reaching a 'mild' increase. I placed the mild in quotes because there is no actual benchmark to gauge if the potassium content in your blood is mild or potentially life-threatening. It all depends on various factors in the body. I shall list down a few foods that are high in potassium that you should watch out for:

- Melons such as cantaloupe and honeydew (watermelon is acceptable)
- Oranges and orange juice
- Winter squash
- Pumpkin
- Bananas
- Prune juice
- Grapefruit juice
- Dried beans – all kinds
- Try to avoid granola bars (even though they are advertised as nutritious) and bran cereals.

Phosphorus

Finally, we have phosphorus. This mineral makes up about 1% of your body weight. That may not seem like a lot but remember that our body consists of a lot of water. For this reason, oxygen makes up 62% of our total body weight, followed by carbon at 18%, hydrogen at 9%, and nitrogen at 3%. But guess which are the next two major elements in the human body?

Calcium at 1.5%.

Phosphorus at 1%.

So, you see, even though phosphorus makes up just 1% of the total body weight, it is still a significant element.

What is it used for?

Let me put it this way. Phosphorus is one of the reasons that you can smile wide. It is the reason your skin and other parts of the body are the way they are and do not just fall on the floor, like the way a piece of cloth might when you drop it. Phosphorus is responsible for forming your teeth and the bones that keep your body structure the way it currently is.

Pretty fantastic. We often nominate calcium as the main element in the formation of teeth and bones but forget the less popular and often overlooked partner element that helps with the same task.

However, the fact that phosphorus keeps our teeth and bones healthy is something people eventually discover. They don't discover that phosphorus also plays an important role in helping the body use fats and carbohydrates. The mineral is truly important for the everyday function of the body.

When kidney problems strike us, we don't need the extra amount of phosphorus. While phosphorus is truly important for our bones and teeth, an excessive amount in the blood can lead to weaker bones. Since most of the food that we eat already includes phosphorus, we will try and avoid anything with a high percentage of the mineral.

Fluids

Water sustains us. After all, 60% of the human adult's body is composed of water. Therefore, you might have heard of popular recommendations on how you should be having about eight glasses of water per day.

There is still a debate on exactly how much water is needed by an individual daily. But the fact remains, we need enough to avoid dehydration and keep the body functioning normally.

When you have kidney disease, you may not need as much fluid as you did before. This is because damaged kidneys do not dispose of extra fluids as well as they should. All the extra fluid in your body could be dangerous. It could cause swelling in various areas, high blood pressure, and heart problems. Fluid can also build up around your lungs, preventing you from breathing normally.

There is no measurement of how much fluid is considered as extra fluid. I strongly suggest that you should visit the doctor and get more information about fluid retention from him or her. The doctor will guide you better and help you understand how much fluids you might require. The thing to understand here is that many of the foods that we eat, including fruits, vegetables, and most soups, have a water content in them as well. Getting to know your kidney's ability to hold on to fluids will help you prepare or plan better meals for yourself.

Chapter Four

EASY AND DELICIOUS RECIPES

*C*ooking and Culinary Units Conversion Chart
       If you can quickly convert measurements of recipes, it will save you a ton of time.

The cooking conversion chart below can act as a quick reference list when you follow any of the cookbook's recipes.

Pork, Beef and Lamb Recipes
   1.   **Full-Flavored Lamb and Winter Squash Tagine with Apricots**
   Time: 50 minutes
   Servings: 6
   Freestyle SmartPoints: 6
   Ingredients:

- 1 pound of lamb shoulders, cubed
- 1 tablespoon of coconut oil
- 1 onion, chopped
- 3 garlic cloves, minced
- 1-inch fresh ginger, grated
- ½ pound of medium-sized winter squash, seeded and cubed
- 2 to 3 cups of beef stock

- ¾ cup of dried apricots
- 1 (14-ounce) can of diced tomatoes
- 1 (14-ounce) can of chickpeas
- 1 teaspoon of salt
- 1 teaspoon of black pepper

Instructions:

- Press "Saute" function on your Instant Pot and add the coconut oil.
- Once the oil is hot, add the onions and cook until brown, stirring occasionally.
- Add the cubed lamb to the Instant Pot and cook until brown on all sides.
- Add the garlic and ginger. Give a good stir.
- Add the cubed squash, beef stock, dried apricots, diced tomatoes, chickpeas, salt, and pepper to the pot.
- Lock the lid and cook at high pressure for 20 minutes.
- When the cooking is done, quick release the pressure and remove the lid.
- Serve and enjoy!

Nutrition information per serving:

- Calories: 446
- Fat: 12.4g
- Carbohydrates: 48.4g
- Dietary Fiber: 13.5g
- Protein: 36g

2. Good Tasting Pork Carnitas (Mexican Pulled Pork)

Time: 1 hour and 20 minutes
Servings: 11
Freestyle SmartPoints: 3
Ingredients:

- 2 ½ pounds of trimmed, boneless pork shoulder, cut into 4 pieces
- 2 tablespoons of olive oil

- 1 cup of chicken broth
- 3 chipotle peppers in adobo sauce
- 2 bay leaves
- 2 tablespoons of garlic powder
- ¼ teaspoon of dry adobo seasoning
- ½ teaspoon of onion powder
- 1 ½ teaspoon of cumin
- ¼ teaspoon of dry oregano
- 2 teaspoons of salt
- 1 teaspoon of black pepper

Instructions:

- Season the pork shoulder with salt and pepper.
- Press "Saute" function and add the olive to the Instant Pot.
- Once the oil is hot, add the pork pieces and cook until brown on all sides, about 5 minutes. Remove and set aside.
- Season the pork with garlic powder, cumin, oregano, and dry adobo seasoning.
- Add the chicken broth, chipotle peppers, bay leaves, and pork to the Instant Pot.
- Lock the lid and cook at high pressure for 80 minutes.
- When the cooking is done, naturally release the pressure and remove the lid.
- Transfer the pork to a cutting board and shred using two forks. Return the shredded pork to the pot and stir into the liquid.
- Remove the bay leaves and adjust the seasoning as needed.
- Serve and enjoy!

Nutrition information per serving:

- Calories: 160
- Fat: 7g
- Carbohydrates: 1g
- Dietary Fiber: 1g
- Protein: 20g

3. Magnificent Beef and Broccoli
Time: 20 minutes

Servings: 6
Freestyle SmartPoints: 3
Beef Ingredients:

- 1 ½ pound of boneless beef chuck roast, thinly sliced
- 4 cups of broccoli florets
- 2 garlic cloves, minced
- ½ teaspoon of fresh ginger, grated
- 1 teaspoon of sesame oil
- 1 teaspoon of salt
- 1 teaspoon of black pepper

Sauce Ingredients:

- 1/3 cup of low-sodium soy sauce
- 2/3 cup of beef broth
- 2 tablespoons of oyster sauce
- 3 tablespoons of brown sugar
- 1 ½ teaspoon of sesame oil
- ¼ teaspoon of red pepper chili flake

Cornstarch Ingredients:

- 2 ½ tablespoons of cornstarch plus 3 tablespoons of water

Instructions:

- Season the beef chuck roast with salt, pepper, and sesame oil.
- Press "Saute" function on your Instant Pot and add the olive to the Instant Pot.
- Once the oil is hot, add the beef and cook for 2 minutes or until brown.
- Add the garlic and ginger and cook for 1 minute or until fragrant, stirring occasionally.
- In a medium bowl, add all the sauce ingredients until well combined. Pour the sauce over the beef.
- Lock the lid and cook at high pressure for 6 minutes.
- Meanwhile, in a bowl, add the broccoli and ¼ cup of water. Microwave for 2 to 3 minutes or until the broccoli is tender.

- When the timer beeps, quick release the pressure and remove the lid.
- Press "Saute" function on your Instant Pot and stir in the cornstarch mixture.
- Add the broccoli florets and cook until the sauce has thickened, stirring occasionally. Adjust the seasoning as needed. Serve and enjoy!

Nutrition information per serving:

- Calories: 475
- Fat: 31.9g
- Carbohydrates: 12.8g
- Protein: 32.8g

4. Remarkable Cajun Chili

Time: 30 minutes
Servings: 8
Freestyle SmartPoints: 4
Ingredients:

- 2 tablespoons of olive oil
- 1 green pepper, chopped
- 1 onion, chopped
- 2 celery ribs, chopped
- 2 garlic cloves, minced
- 1 pound of ground beef
- 2 links Andouille Sausage, sliced
- 7-ounces of raw shrimp, peeled and deveined
- 1 tablespoon of parsley, freshly chopped
- 2 ½ tablespoons of Cajun seasoning
- 1 (14-ounce) can of crushed tomatoes
- 1 (14.5-ounce) can of fire roasted tomatoes
- 1 (15-ounce) can of red kidney beans, drained and rinsed
- 2 tablespoons of tomato paste
- 1 teaspoon of salt
- 2 bay leaves

Instructions:

- Press "Saute" function and add 1 tablespoon of olive oil to your Instant Pot.
- Once the oil is hot, add the green pepper, onion, celery, and garlic. Cook for 4 minutes or until softened, stirring occasionally.
- Add the remaining 1 tablespoon of olive oil and ground beef. Cook until brown, stirring frequently.
- Add the sausage and cook for 5 minutes or until brown, stirring occasionally.
- Add the shrimp and remaining ingredients to your Instant Pot. Stir until well combined.
- Lock the lid and cook at high pressure for 10 minutes.
- When the cooking is done, naturally release the pressure and remove the lid.
- Press "Saute" function on your Instant Pot and cook for 5 to 7 minutes or until the chili has thickened, stirring occasionally. Serve and enjoy!

Nutrition information per serving:

- Calories: 344
- Fat: 16.4g
- Carbohydrates: 24g
- Dietary Fiber: 6.4g
- Protein: 27.6g

5. Phenomenal Chipotle Chili
Time: 40 minutes
Servings: 4
Freestyle SmartPoints: 5
Ingredients:

- 1 pound of ground beef
- 1 tablespoon of coconut oil
- 1 large onion, finely chopped
- 6 garlic cloves, minced
- 1 teaspoon of chipotle chili powder
- 1 tablespoon of red chili powder
- 1 teaspoon of oregano

- 1 teaspoon of cumin powder
- 2 chipotle chilies in adobo sauce, roughly chopped
- 2 cups of fresh tomatoes, chopped
- 1 cup of dried kidney beans, soaked overnight
- 1 cup of water or beef broth
- 1 teaspoon of salt
- 1 teaspoon of black pepper

Topping ingredients:

- Sliced avocados
- Crushed nachos
- Lime wedges
- Sour cream
- Cilantro
- Shredded cheddar cheese

Instructions:

- Press "Saute" function on your Instant Pot and add the coconut oil.
- Once the oil is hot and ready, add the ground beef and cook until brown, stirring occasionally.
- Add the onions and garlic. Cook until softened, stirring occasionally.
- Add the remaining ingredients to your Instant Pot and stir until well combined.
- Lock the lid and cook at high pressure for 30 minutes.
- When the cooking is done, naturally release the pressure and remove the lid.
- Stir in the chili and adjust the seasoning as needed.
- Spoon the chili into serving bowls and add desired toppings. Serve and enjoy!

Nutrition information per serving:

- Calories: 459
- Fat: 26g
- Carbohydrates: 25.4g

- Protein: 28g

6. **Homemade Hamburger Helper**

Time: 10 minutes
S rvings: 6
Freestyle SmartPoints: 7
Ingredients:

- 1 pound of ground beef
- 2 cups of beef broth
- 2 cups of elbow macaroni
- 1 cup of heavy cream
- 2 cups of shredded cheddar cheese
- ½ cup of shredded American cheese
- 1 tablespoon of onion powder
- 1 tablespoon of garlic powder

Instructions:

- Press "Saute' function on your Instant Pot and add the ground beef and seasonings. Cook until the meat is brown, stirring occasionally.
- Add the beef broth, elbow macaroni, and heavy cream to your Instant Pot.
- Lock the lid and cook at high pressure for 4 minutes.
- When the cooking is done, quick release the pressure and remove the lid.
- Stir in the cheddar cheese and American cheese. Continue to cook and stir until all the cheese has melted.
- Serve and enjoy!

Nutrition information per serving:

- Calories: 992
- Fat: 61g
- Carbohydrates: 61g
- Dietary Fiber: 2g
- Protein: 47g

7. **Famous Spaghetti**

Time: 15 minutes
Servings: 6
Freestyle SmartPoints: 5
Ingredients:

- 1 pound of lean ground beef
- ½ teaspoon of salt
- ½ teaspoon of garlic powder
- ½ teaspoon of onion powder
- ½ teaspoon of Italian seasoning
- 1 pound of spaghetti noodles, break in half
- 1 (24-ounce) jar of spaghetti sauce
- 4 ½ cup of water
- 1 (14.5-ounce) can of diced tomatoes

Instructions:

- Press "Saute" function on your Instant Pot and add the ground beef.
- Add the salt, garlic powder, onion powder, and Italian seasoning. Cook until the ground beef is completely brown, stirring occasionally.
- Turn off "Saute' function on your Instant Pot and discard any excess grease from the beef if necessary.
- Add the spaghetti noodles, spaghetti sauce, water, and diced tomatoes to your Instant Pot.
- Lock the lid and cook at high pressure for 8 minutes.
- When the cooking is done, quick release the pressure and remove the lid
- Stir the spaghetti and adjust the seasoning as needed. Serve and enjoy!

Nutrition information per serving:

- Calories: 689
- Fat: 7.7g
- Carbohydrates: 116.9g
- Dietary Fiber: 4.2g

- Protein: 38.9g

8.   Tempting Beef Short Ribs

Time: 1 hour and 20 minutes
Servings: 10
Freestyle SmartPoints: 9
Ingredients:

- 4 pounds of boneless beef short ribs
- 2 tablespoons of olive oil
- 1 large onion, chopped
- 2 shallots, finely chopped
- 3 garlic cloves, minced
- 3 large carrots, chopped
- 1 sprig of rosemary
- 2 sprigs of thyme, leaves removed
- 1 cup of red wine
- 1 cup of chicken broth
- 3 tablespoons of balsamic vinegar
- 2 teaspoons of salt
- 1 teaspoon of black pepper

Instructions:

- Season the ribs with salt and pepper.
- Press "Saute" function on your Instant Pot and add 1 tablespoon of olive oil.
- Add the ribs to your Instant Pot and sear for 6 to 8 minutes.
- Flip the ribs and cook for 5 minutes or until brown.
- Once the meat is brown, transfer to a plate and add the remaining tablespoon of olive oil.
- Add the onions, shallots, garlic, and carrots to your Instant Pot and cook until soft.
- Add the red wine, chicken broth, and balsamic vinegar to your Instant Pot. Stir until well combined.
- Return the beef short ribs to your Instant Pot and top with rosemary.
- Lock the lid and cook at high pressure for 45 minutes.

- When the cooking is done, naturally release the pressure and remove the lid.
- Transfer the ribs to a serving platter.
- Press "Saute" function and bring the broth to a boil. Cook until half of the liquid has reduced and thickened, stirring occasionally. Sprinkle with thyme leaves
- Pour the sauce over the ribs. Serve and enjoy!

Nutrition information per serving:

- Calories: 407
- Fat: 14.3g
- Carbohydrates: 5.9g
- Dietary Fiber: 0.9g
- Protein: 56.2g

Chicken, Turkey and Duck Recipes
1. Summer Italian Chicken
Time: 30 minutes
Servings: 8
Freestyle SmartPoints: 3
Ingredients:

- 8 boneless, skinless chicken thighs
- 2 tablespoons of avocado oil
- 1 onion, chopped
- 2 medium carrots, chopped
- ½ pounds of cremini mushrooms stemmed and quartered
- 4 garlic cloves, minced
- 1 tablespoon of tomato paste
- 2 cups of cherry tomatoes
- ½ cup of green olives pitted
- ½ cup of fresh basil leaves, thinly sliced
- ¼ cup of Italian parsley, chopped
- 1 teaspoon of salt
- 1 teaspoon of black pepper

Instructions:

- Season the chicken thighs with salt and pepper.
- Press "Saute" function on your Instant Pot and add the avocado oil.
- Once the oil is hot, add the onions, carrots, and mushrooms. Cook for 3 to 5 minutes or until the vegetables have softened.
- Stir in the garlic and tomato paste. Cook for 30 seconds or until fragrant.
- Add the chicken, cherry tomatoes, green olives. Stir until well combined.
- Lock the lid and cook at high pressure for 8 minutes.
- When the cooking is done, quick release the pressure and remove the lid.
- Stir in the basil leaves and parsley. Adjust the seasoning as needed.
- Serve and enjoy!

Nutrition information per serving:

- Calories: 318
- Fat: 11.9g
- Carbohydrates: 7.1g
- Dietary Fiber: 2g
- Protein: 44.2g

2. Delectable Chicken Enchiladas
Time: 50 minutes
Servings: 4
Freestyle SmartPoints: 3
Ingredients:

- 1 pound of boneless, skinless chicken thighs
- 2 cups of ancho chili sauce
- ½ cup of onions, chopped
- 12 corn tortillas
- 3 tablespoons of olive oil
- ½ cup of crumbled queso fresco
- 2 cups of shredded Monterey Jack cheese
- 1 teaspoon of salt
- 1 teaspoon of black pepper

Instructions:

- Add the chicken thighs and ancho chili sauce to your Instant Pot.
- Lock the lid and cook at high pressure for 10 minutes.
- When the cooking is done, naturally release the pressure for 10 minutes and quick release any remaining pressure.
- Remove the lid and transfer the chicken to a large bowl. Shred the chicken using forks. Stir in 2/3 cup of the ancho chili sauce.
- Chop the onions and put into a small bowl.
- Preheat your oven to 350 degrees Fahrenheit.
- Place tortillas on a baking sheet and lightly brush with olive oil.
- Place inside your oven and bake for 3 minutes or until warm. Remove from the oven.
- Spoon ½ cup of the warm ancho chili sauce into a baking dish.
- Working one-by-one, lightly coat each tortilla with the sauce and generously add the shredded chicken and onions on the tortilla.
- Sprinkle shredded Monterey Jack cheese over the chicken and onion.
- Wrap the tortilla and repeat until all the tortillas are used up.
- Once all the tortillas are prepared, generously pour leftover ancho chili sauce over them and sprinkle remaining cheese over the enchiladas.
- Place inside your oven and bake for 8 to 10 minutes or until warmed through.
- Sprinkle crumbled queso fresco over the enchiladas. Serve and enjoy!

Nutrition information per serving:

- Calories: 695
- Fat: 38g
- Carbohydrates: 67g
- Protein: 51g

3. **Finger Licking Chicken Marsala**
Time: 40 minutes
Servings: 4

Freestyle SmartPoints: 4
Ingredients:

- 5 boneless, skinless chicken breasts, halved or thinly sliced
- ½ cup of all-purpose flour
- 3 tablespoons of butter
- 3 tablespoons of olive oil
- 1 cup of mushrooms, stemmed and halved
- 1 shallot, thinly sliced
- 3 garlic cloves, minced
- 2/3 cup of marsala wine
- 2/3 cup of chicken stock
- ½ cup of heavy cream
- 1 teaspoon of garlic powder
- 1 teaspoon of salt
- 1 teaspoon of black pepper

Instructions:

- Add the flour on a shallow plate and dredge the chicken breasts in the flour, shake off any excess flour.
- Press "Saute" function on your Instant Pot and add the 2 tablespoons of oil and 2 tablespoons of butter.
- Once the butter is melted, working in batches, add the chicken breasts and cook on both sides until golden. Set the cooked chicken aside.
- Add the remaining tablespoons of oil and butter to your Instant Pot.
- Add the mushrooms, shallots, and garlic. Cook for 5 minutes or until tender, stirring occasionally. Season with salt and pepper.
- Add the marsala wine and chicken stock to your Instant Pot. Stir until well combined. Lay the chicken on top of the mushrooms.
- Lock the lid and cook at high pressure for 10 minutes.
- When the cooking is done, naturally release the pressure for 5 minutes and quick release any remaining pressure. Remove the lid. Remove the chicken and set aside.
- Press "Saute" function and stir in the heavy cream. Stir until

well combined. Cook for 5 minutes or until thickened, stirring occasionally.
- Return the chicken back to the pot and stir until well coated. Serve and enjoy!

Nutrition information per serving:

- Calories: 622
- Fat: 35g
- Carbohydrates: 23g
- Dietary Fiber: 1g
- Protein: 41g

4. Award Winning Turkey Chili
Time: 18 minutes
Servings: 8
Freestyle SmartPoints: 3
Ingredients:

- 1 ½ pound of ground turkey
- 8 bacon slices, chopped
- 1 (15-ounce) can of pinto beans, rinsed and drained
- 1 (15-ounce) can of black beans, rinsed and drained
- 1 (15-ounce) can of diced tomatoes, rinsed and drained
- 1 (6-ounce) can of tomato paste
- 1 small red onion, chopped
- 1 red bell pepper, chopped
- 1 orange bell pepper, chopped
- 1 jalapeno, minced
- 2 cups of chicken stock
- 1 tablespoon of dried oregano
- 1 teaspoon of ground cumin
- 2 teaspoons of salt
- 1 teaspoon of black pepper
- 1 teaspoon of smoked paprika
- 2 tablespoons of chili powder
- 1 tablespoon of Worcestershire sauce
- 1 tablespoon of garlic, minced

Topping Ingredients:

- Sour cream
- Cilantro
- Shredded cheese

Instructions:

- Press "Saute" function on your Instant Pot and add the bacon. Cook until brown and crispy, stirring occasionally. Remove the bacon and set on a paper towel-lined plate. Add the onions and peppers and cook until softened, stirring occasionally.
- Add the ground turkey and cook until browned, stirring occasionally.
- Add the remaining ingredients and cooked bacon. Stir until well combined.
- Lock the lid and cook at high pressure for 18 minutes.
- When the cooking is done, naturally release the pressure for 15 minutes and quick release any remaining pressure. Remove the lid.
- Ladle the chili into serving bowls and top with desired toppings. Serve and enjoy!

Nutrition information per serving:

- Calories: 286
- Fat: 11.7g
- Carbohydrates: 19.7g
- Dietary Fiber: 6.3g
- Protein: 26.3

5. Tantalizing Beer-And-Mustard Pulled Turkey

Time: 1 hour
Servings: 4
Freestyle SmartPoints: 6
Ingredients:

- 2 (1 ½ pound) bone-in, skinless turkey thighs
- 1 (12-ounce) bottle of dark beer

- ½ teaspoon of garlic powder
- 1 teaspoon of black pepper
- 1 teaspoon of salt
- 1 teaspoon of dry mustard
- 2 teaspoons of ground coriander
- 2 tablespoons of brown sugar
- 2 tablespoons of apple cider vinegar
- 1 tablespoon of mustard
- 1 tablespoon of canned tomato paste

Instructions:

- In a bowl, add the coriander, dry mustard, salt, black pepper, and garlic powder. Mix well.
- Rub and coat the spice mixture over the turkey thighs.
- Add the turkey thighs to your Instant Pot and add in the beer.
- Lock the lid and cook at high pressure for 45 minutes.
- When the cooking is done, quick release the pressure and remove the lid.
- Transfer the turkey thighs to a plate and shred using forks. Set aside.
- Press "Saute" function on your Instant Pot and allow the liquid to simmer until reduced to about half.
- Stir in the brown sugar, apple cider vinegar, mustard, and tomato paste until smooth. Cook for 1 minute, stirring occasionally.
- Return the turkey and give a good stir.

Nutrition information per serving:

- Calories: 406
- Fat: 20.1g
- Carbohydrates: 3g
- Dietary Fiber: 0g
- Protein: 44.7g

6. **Extraordinary Honey Garlic Chicken**
Time: 25 minutes
Servings: 4

Freestyle SmartPoints: 9
Ingredients:

- 4 to 6 bone-in, skinless chicken thighs
- 1/3 cup of honey
- 4 garlic cloves, minced
- ½ cup of low-sodium soy sauce
- ½ cup of sugar-free ketchup
- ½ teaspoon of dried oregano
- 2 tablespoons of parsley, chopped
- 1 tablespoon of sesame seed oil
- 1 teaspoon of salt
- 1 teaspoon of black pepper
- ½ tablespoon of toasted sesame seeds, for garnish

Instructions:

- In a bowl, add the honey, garlic, soy sauce, ketchup, oregano, and parsley Mix until well combined and set aside.
- Season the chicken thighs with salt and pepper.
- Press "Saute" function and add the sesame oil.
- Once the oil is hot, add the chicken thighs and cook for 3 minutes on both sides.
- Add the honey garlic sauce to your Instant Pot.
- Lock the lid and cook at high pressure for 20 minutes.
- When the cooking is done, naturally release the pressure for 5 minutes and quick release any remaining pressure.
- Transfer the chicken to serving plate and spoon the sauce over. Serve and enjoy!

Nutrition information per serving:

- Calories: 360
- Fat: 10g
- Carbohydrates: 35g
- Dietary Fiber: 6g
- Protein: 32g

7. **Refreshing Duck Confit**

Time: 2 hours
Servings: 4
Freestyle SmartPoints: 3
Ingredients:

- 4 duck legs
- 2 tablespoons of olive oil
- 1 tablespoon of salt
- 4 sprigs fresh thyme
- 4 garlic cloves, crushed
- 2 bay leaves, torn in half
- ¼ teaspoon of black peppercorns, crushed
- ¼ teaspoon of allspice berries, crushed

Instructions:

- Season the duck legs with salt, bay leaves, peppercorns, and allspice.
- Press "Saute" function on your Instant Pot and add the olive oil.
- Once the oil is hot, add the duck legs and cook until golden brown on both sides.
- Add the garlic and thyme on top of the duck.
- Lock the lid and cook at high pressure for 40 minutes. You don't need to add any additional liquid as the duck legs contain enough moisture to create steam.
- When the timer beeps, quick release the pressure and remove the lid. Flip the duck legs over.
- Lock the lid and cook at high pressure for 30 minutes.
- When the cooking is done, naturally release the pressure and remove the lid.
- Remove the duck legs and allow to cool.
- Serve and enjoy!

Nutrition information per serving:

- Calories: 194
- Fat: 11.5g
- Carbohydrates: 0g
- Dietary Fiber: 0g

- Protein: 21.8g

8. Exquisite Orange Duck and Gravy

Time: 1 hour and 30 minutes
Servings: 4
Freestyle SmartPoints: 5
Ingredients:

- 4 duck legs
- 2 tablespoons of avocado oil
- 1 yellow onion, chopped
- 1 celery rib, chopped
- 1 large carrot, chopped
- 8 garlic cloves, crushed
- 1 tablespoon of tomato paste
- ½ cup of chicken stock
- 1 teaspoon of orange zest
- ¼ cup of orange juice
- 2 tablespoons of Italian parsley, chopped
- 1 dried bay leaf
- 1 fresh thyme sprig
- ½ teaspoon of herbes de Provence
- 1 teaspoon of salt
- 1 teaspoon of black pepper

Instructions:

- In a small bowl, add the salt, black pepper, and herbes de Provence. Mix well.
- Sprinkle the seasonings over the duck legs.
- Press "Saute" function on your Instant Pot and add 1 tablespoon of avocado oil.
- Add the onions, celery, and carrots. Cook for 3 to 5 minutes or until the vegetables has softened, stirring occasionally.
- Add the garlic cloves and tomato paste. Cook for 30 seconds or until fragrant, stirring occasionally. Pour in the chicken stock to the pot.
- Stir in the orange juice, orange zest, parsley, bay leaf, and thyme.

Turn off "Saute" function. Place the seasoned dug legs on top of the vegetables.

- Lock the lid and cook at high pressure for 45 minutes.
- When the cooking is done, naturally release the pressure for 20 minutes and remove the lid.
- Carefully remove the duck legs and discard the thyme sprig and bay leaf.
- Use an immersion blender to puree the contents of the Instant Pot until smooth and thick. Adjust the seasoning as needed.
- Heat a large cast-iron skillet over medium-high heat. Once the skillet is hot, add 1 tablespoon of avocado oil and duck legs. Cook for 2 to 3 minutes on both sides or until golden brown and crispy.
- Place the duck legs onto serving plates and spoon the gravy over. Serve!

Nutrition information per serving: Calories: 183, Fat: 5.6g, Carbohydrates: 9.5g, Dietary Fiber: 1.8g, Protein: 23.2g

Fish and Seafood Recipes

1. **Gorgeous Lemon-Shrimp Risotto with Vegetables and Parmesan**

Time: 25 minutes
Servings: 4
Freestyle SmartPoints: 4
Ingredients:

- 1 ½ cup of Arborio rice
- 1 pound of shrimp, peeled and deveined
- ½ cup of Parmigiano-Reggiano, shredded
- 2 teaspoons of olive oil
- 1 cup of fresh spinach
- 1 bunch of asparagus, sliced
- 3 ½ cup of chicken stock
- ½ cup of dry white wine
- 3 garlic cloves, minced
- ½ white onion, chopped
- 1 tablespoon of parsley, chopped
- ½ lemon, juiced
- 1 tablespoon of butter

- 1 teaspoon of salt
- 1 teaspoon of black pepper

Instructions:

- Press "Saute" function on your Instant Pot and add the olive oil.
- Once the oil is hot and ready, add the asparagus and cook for 3 minutes or until softened, stirring constantly. Once done, remove the asparagus.
- Add the onions and garlic and cook until fragrant, stirring occasionally.
- Add the butter and rice to your Instant Pot. Stir for 1 to 2 minutes or until the rice is coated in butter.
- Stir in the white wine, chicken stock, and cheese. Season with salt and black pepper. Lock the lid and cook at high pressure for 8 minutes.
- When the cooking is done, quick release the pressure and remove the lid.
- Press "Saute" function and add the shrimp, spinach, and asparagus.
- Cook for about 4 minutes or until the shrimp is pink and the spinach has wilted, stirring occasionally. Turn off "Saute" function. Drizzle with fresh lemon juice and sprinkle with parsley. Serve and enjoy!

Nutrition information per serving:

- Calories: 440
- Fat: 12g
- Carbohydrates: 48g
- Dietary Fiber: 4g
- Protein: 29g

2. Nourishing Garlic Butter Salmon and Asparagus

Time: 9 minutes
Servings: 3
Freestyle SmartPoints: 4
Ingredients:

- 1 pound of salmon fillets, cut into 3 equal pieces
- 1 pound of asparagus, cut into bite-sized pieces
- ¼ cup of lemon juice
- 3 tablespoons of butter
- 1 ½ tablespoon of garlic, minced
- 1 teaspoon of salt
- ¼ teaspoon of red pepper flakes
- 2 cups of water

Instructions:

- Lay 3 large pieces of foil on a flat surface.
- Place 1 salmon piece on each foil.
- Spread ½ tablespoon of garlic on each piece of salmon.
- Divide and place the asparagus equally between the three salmon pieces.
- Sprinkle salt and red pepper flakes on top of each salmon fillet.
- Add 1 tablespoon of butter on each salmon fillet.
- Tightly wrap the foil and make sure no steam can escape.
- Add 2 cups of water and a trivet to your Instant Pot.
- Place the foil packets on top of the trivet.
- Lock the lid and press "Steam" function and set for 4 minutes.
- When the cooking is done, quick release the pressure and remove the lid.
- Remove the foil packets and unopen. Transfer the contents to a plate.
- Serve and enjoy!

Nutrition information per serving:

- Calories: 343
- Fat: 21.2g
- Carbohydrates: 8.9g
- Dietary Fiber: 3.8g
- Protein: 33.2g

3. Pleasant Fish and Potato Chowder

Time: 30 minutes
Servings: 8

Freestyle SmartPoints: 4
Ingredients:

- 2 ½ cups of fish stock or water
- 1 ½ pounds of tilapia, cut into bite-sized pieces
- 1 pound of potatoes, chopped
- 1 cup of celery, chopped
- 1 cup of onions, chopped
- 6 bacon slices, chopped
- 1 ½ cup of unsweetened coconut cream
- 3 tablespoons of butter
- ½ teaspoon of garlic powder
- 1 teaspoon of salt
- 1 teaspoon of black pepper

Instructions:

- Press "Saute" function on your Instant Pot and add the bacon. Cook the bacon until brown and crispy.
- Remove the bacon and set aside.
- Add the butter, onions, and celery. Cook until the onions have softened, stirring frequently.
- Add the fish stock, tilapia pieces, salt, pepper, garlic powder, bacon and coconut cream to your Instant Pot. Give a good stir.
- Lock the lid and cook at high pressure for 10 minutes.
- When the cooking is done, naturally release the pressure and remove the lid.
- Use a potato masher to mash the potatoes until broken down. You can leave chunks if you prefer.
- Serve and enjoy!

Nutrition information per serving:

- Calories: 348
- Fat: 22.5g
- Carbohydrates: 13.3g
- Dietary Fiber: 2.9g
- Protein: 25g

4. Soy-Free Asian Salmon

Time: 7 minutes
Servings: 2
Freestyle SmartPoints: 3
Ingredients:

- 2 salmon fillets
- 1 tablespoon of coconut oil
- 1 tablespoon of brown sugar
- 3 tablespoons of coconut aminos
- 2 tablespoons of maple syrup
- 1 tablespoon of parsley, chopped
- 1 teaspoon of paprika
- ¼ teaspoon of ginger
- 1 teaspoon of sesame seeds
- 1 teaspoon of salt
- 1 teaspoon of black pepper

Instructions:

- Press "Saute" function on your Instant Pot and add the coconut oil.
- Once the oil is hot, add the brown sugar and stir until the sugar has dissolved.
- Stir in the paprika, ginger, coconut aminos, and maple syrup.
- Add the salmon fillets to your Instant Pot and season with salt and pepper.
- Lock the lid and cook at low pressure for 2 minutes.
- When the cooking is done, naturally release the pressure for 5 minutes and quick release any remaining pressure.
- Remove the lid and transfer the salmon fillets to a plate.
- Spoon and pour some of the broth over the salmon.
- Sprinkle the fillets with sesame seeds and garnish with parsley
- Serve and enjoy!

Nutrition information per serving:

- Calories: 378
- Fat: 17.8g

- Carbohydrates: 20.8g
- Dietary Fiber: 0g
- Protein: 34.5g

5. Traditional Lemon Garlic Salmon

Time: 10 minutes
Servings: 2
Freestyle SmartPoints: 2
Ingredients:

- 1 ½ pounds of frozen salmon fillets
- ¼ cup of lemon juice
- ¾ cup of fish stock or water
- 1 lemon, thinly sliced
- 1 tablespoon of coconut oil
- 2 tablespoons of mixed herbs
- 1 teaspoon of garlic powder
- 1 teaspoon of salt
- 1 teaspoon of black pepper

Instructions:

- Add the lemon juice, fish stock, and mixed herbs to your Instant Pot.
- Place a steamer rack in Instant Pot.
- Drizzle the salmon fillets with coconut oil and season with garlic powder, salt, and black pepper.
- Place the salmon on the steamer rack and place lemon slices on top.
- Lock the lid and cook at high pressure for 7 minutes.
- When the cooking is done, quick release the pressure and remove the lid.
- Serve and enjoy!

Nutrition information per serving:

- Calories: 539
- Fat: 28.8g
- Carbohydrates: 3.3g

- Dietary Fiber: 0.9g
- Protein: 58.5g

6. Decorated Salmon, Broccoli, and Potatoes

Time: 6 minutes
Servings: 2
Freestyle SmartPoints: 2
Ingredients:

- 2 (4-ounce) salmon fillet
- 1 medium head of broccoli, chopped into florets
- 1 potato, chopped into cubes
- 1 shallot, chopped
- 2 garlic cloves, minced
- 3 tablespoons of butter
- 1 tablespoon of coconut oil
- ½ cup of fish stock
- 1 tablespoon of parsley, chopped
- 1 teaspoon of salt
- 1 teaspoon of black pepper

Instructions:

- Drizzle the coconut oil over the salmon fillet and season with salt and pepper
- Press "Saute" function on your Instant Pot and add the butter.
- Once the butter has melted, add the shallot and cook until softened, stirring occasionally.
- Add the garlic and cook for 1 minute or until fragrant.
- Add the broccoli, potatoes, and parsley to your Instant Pot. Cook for 2 minutes, stirring occasionally.
- Add ½ cup of fish stock and a steaming rack to your Instant Pot.
- Place the salmon fillets on top of the rack.
- Lock the lid and cook at high pressure for 4 minutes.
- When the cooking is done, naturally release the pressure and remove the lid.
- Transfer the salmon fillet to a plate along with the broccoli and potato mixture.

- Serve and enjoy!

Nutrition information per serving:

- Calories: 467
- Fat: 31.8g
- Carbohydrates: 21.4g
- Dietary Fiber: 3.1g
- Protein: 27.1g

7. **Wonderful in Taste Fish Taco Bowls**

Time: 15 minutes
Servings: 4
Freestyle SmartPoints: 3
Fish Ingredients:

- 3 (6-ounce) cod fillets
- 1 tablespoon of olive oil
- ½ teaspoon of salt
- ½ teaspoon of black pepper
- 1 cup of water

Slaw Ingredients:

- ½ cup of green cabbage, grated
- 1 large carrot, peeled and grated
- 2 tablespoons of fresh orange juice
- 2 dashes of sriracha sauce
- ¼ cup of cilantro, freshly chopped
- ¼ cup of low-fat mayonnaise
- 1 medium avocado, peeled and diced
- 2 Roma tomatoes, chopped
- ½ large lime, juice
- 1 teaspoon of ground cumin
- 1 teaspoon of garlic salt

Instructions:

- In a large bowl, add all the slaw ingredients and stir until well combined.
- Add 1 cup of water and a trivet to your Instant Pot.
- Place a steamer basket on top of the trivet.
- Season the cod fillets with salt and pepper and drizzle olive oil.
- Place the cod fillets onto steamer basket.
- Lock the lid and cook at high pressure for 3 minutes.
- When the cooking is done, quick release the pressure and remove the lid.
- Distribute the slaw into serving bowls and add the cod fillet.
- Serve and enjoy!

Nutrition information per serving:

- Calories: 284
- Fat: 19.1g
- Carbohydrates: 13.4g
- Dietary Fiber: 4.8g
- Protein: 17g

8.   Wholesome Clam Chowder

Time: 30 minutes
Servings: 6
Freestyle SmartPoints: 5
Ingredients:

- 3 (6.5-ounce) cans of chopped clams, juice reserved
- 4 slices of bacon, chopped
- 3 tablespoons of butter
- 1 onion, chopped
- 2 celery stalks, chopped
- 1 ½ pounds of potatoes, chopped
- 1 1/3 cup of heavy cream
- 1 tablespoon of cornstarch
- ¼ teaspoon of dried thyme
- 1 garlic clove, minced
- 1 ½ teaspoon of salt
- ¼ teaspoon of black pepper

Instructions:

- Press "Saute" function and add the chopped bacon to your Instant Pot. Cook the bacon until no more fat, but not crispy.
- Add the butter, onion, celery, and thyme. Cook for 4 minutes or until the onions are translucent, stirring occasionally.
- Add the garlic, salt, and black pepper. Cook for 1 minute or until fragrant, stirring frequently.
- Stir in the potatoes and clam juice.
- Lock the lid and cook at high pressure for 5 minutes.
- When the cooking is done, quick release the pressure and remove the lid.
- Use a potato masher and mash the potatoes.
- Press" Saute" function and stir in the clams and heavy cream.
- Add the cornstarch and cook until thickened. Adjust the seasoning as needed.
- Serve and enjoy!

Nutrition information per serving:

- Calories: 386
- Fat: 25.7g
- Carbohydrates: 32.7g
- Dietary Fiber: 4.9g
- Protein: 8.8g

Vegan and Vegetarian Recipes
1. Indian-Inspired Pickled Potatoes
Time: 15 minutes
Servings: 4
Freestyle SmartPoints: 3
Ingredients:

- 5 potatoes, boiled and cubed
- 4 tablespoons of olive oil
- 1 bay leaf
- 5 cloves
- 1 tablespoon of coriander seeds, pounded
- 1 tablespoon of cumin seeds

- 1 tablespoon of mango pickle
- 2 teaspoons of dried fenugreek leaves
- 1 teaspoon of dry pomegranate powder
- ½ teaspoon of turmeric powder
- ½ teaspoon of red chili powder
- 1 teaspoon of salt

Instructions:

- Press "Saute" function on your Instant Pot and add 2 tablespoons of olive oil.
- Once the oil is hot, add the cumin seeds, coriander seeds, cloves, and bay leaf. Allow simmering for a few seconds.
- Add the dry spices and mix them well.
- Add the remaining 2 tablespoons of olive oil and pickle. Stir the mixture well.
- Add the potatoes and coat them with the spice mixture.
- Lock the lid and cook at high pressure for 2 minutes.
- When the cooking is done, quick release the pressure and remove the lid.
- Serve and enjoy!

Nutrition information per serving:

- Calories: 304
- Fat: 14.3g
- Carbohydrates: 41.8g
- Dietary Fiber: 6.4g
- Protein: 4.5g

2.   Satisfying Vegan Quinoa Burrito Bowls
Time: 25 minutes
Servings: 4
Freestyle SmartPoints: 3
Ingredients:

- 1 teaspoon of olive oil
- ½ red onion, chopped
- 1 sweet bell pepper, chopped

- 1 cup of quinoa, rinsed well
- 1 cup of salsa
- 1 cup of water
- 1 (15-ounce) can of black beans, drained and rinsed
- ½ teaspoon of salt
- 1 teaspoon of ground cumin

Topping ingredients (optional):

- Avocado slices
- Guacamole
- Fresh cilantro
- Green onions, chopped
- Salsa
- Lime wedges
- Lettuce, shredded

Instructions:

- Press "Saute" function on your Instant Pot and add the olive oil.
- Once the oil is hot, add the onions and pepper and cook for 5 minutes or until softened, stirring constantly.
- Add the cumin and salt and cook for an additional minute.
- Turn off "Saute" function on your Instant Pot.
- Add the quinoa, salsa, water, and black beans to your Instant Pot. Stir until well combined.
- Lock the lid and cook at low pressure for 12 minutes.
- When the cooking is done, naturally release the pressure and remove the lid.
- Fluff the quinoa with a fork and spoon into serving bowls.
- Top with your desired toppings.
- Serve and enjoy!

Nutrition information per serving:

- Calories: 562
- Fat: 5.5g
- Carbohydrates: 101.2g
- Dietary Fiber: 20.9g

- Protein: 30.4g

3. **Signature Curried Chickpea Stuffed Acorn Squash**

Time: 30 minutes
Servings: 2
Freestyle SmartPoints: 5
Ingredients:

- 2 cups of chickpeas, soaked in water for 30 minutes
- ¼ cup of brown rice washed and soaked in water for 30 minutes
- 2 cups of vegetable stock
- 1 small acorn squash, halved and deseeded
- 1 tablespoon of olive oil
- ½ teaspoon of cumin seeds
- ½ cup of red onions, chopped
- 4 garlic cloves, minced
- ½-inch ginger, minced
- 1 green chili, minced
- ¼ teaspoon of turmeric
- ½ teaspoon of garam masala
- ½ teaspoon of dry mango powder amchur
- 2 tomatoes, chopped
- ½ teaspoon of fresh lime juice
- 1 cup of rainbow chard or spinach, chopped
- ½ teaspoon of salt
- ¼ teaspoon of cayenne pepper

Instructions:

- Add the olive oil to your Instant Pot and press "Saute" setting.
- Add the cumin seeds and cook for 1 minute or until fragrant, stirring frequently.
- Add the onions, garlic, ginger, and chili. Cook for 5 minutes or until translucent, stirring frequently.
- Add the seasoning and stir for a couple of seconds.
- Add the tomatoes, lime juice, and rainbow chard or spinach. Cook for 5 minutes, stirring occasionally.
- Add the remaining ingredients except for the acorn squash to your Instant Pot and stir until well combined.

- Place a steamer basket or a trivet to your Instant Pot and place the acorn squash on top. Lock the lid and cook at high pressure for 17 minutes.
- When the cooking is done, naturally release the pressure and remove the lid.
- Carefully remove the steamer basket and stir the chickpea rice stew.
- Fill the squash with the chickpea rice mixture. Serve and enjoy!

Nutrition information per serving:

- Calories: 518
- Fat: 8g
- Carbohydrates: 97g
- Protein: 20g

4. **Terrific Vegan Sloppy Joes**
Time: 30 minutes
Servings: 8
Freestyle SmartPoints: 3
Ingredients:

- 1 cup of green/brown lentils
- 1 cup of red lentils
- 3 cups of water
- 1 large onion, chopped
- 1 red bell pepper, chopped
- 1 tablespoon of olive oil
- 2 tablespoons of apple cider vinegar
- 2 tablespoons of maple syrup
- 1 (28-ounce) can of crushed tomatoes
- 3 tablespoons of tomato paste
- 2 tablespoons of vegan Worcestershire sauce
- 1 teaspoon of salt
- 1 tablespoon of ground cumin
- 1 teaspoon of dried oregano

Instructions:

- Press "Saute" function on your Instant Pot and add the olive oil.
- Once the oil is hot, add the onion, bell pepper, and salt. Cook for 3 minutes or until softened, stirring frequently.
- Add the cumin and oregano and cook for 1 minute.
- Add the tomato paste and cook for 2 minutes, stirring to coat.
- Add the remaining ingredients and stir until well combined.
- Lock the lid and cook at high pressure for 13 minutes.
- When the cooking is done, allow for a natural release and remove the lid.
- Stir everything again and adjust the seasoning as needed.
- Serve over toasted hamburger buns.

Nutrition information per serving:

- Calories: 259
- Fat: 3.1g
- Carbohydrates: 47.3g
- Dietary Fiber: 5.4g
- Protein: 14.4g

5. Mexican-Style Corn on the Cob with Hemp-Lime Sauce
Time: 30 minutes
Servings: 4
Freestyle SmartPoints: 2
Ingredients:

- 4 ear corns, shucked and rinsed
- ½ cup of unsweetened coconut milk
- 2 tablespoons of hemp hearts
- 2 tablespoons of nutritional yeast
- 1 tablespoon of all-purpose flour
- 1 garlic clove, peeled
- ¼ teaspoon of cayenne pepper
- ¼ teaspoon of salt
- 1 tablespoon of fresh lime juice

Instructions:

- Place a trivet or a steaming basket inside your Instant Pot.

- Add 1 ½ cup of water and a trivet or steamer basket in your Instant Pot.
- Lock the lid and cook at high pressure for 4 minutes.
- When the cooking is done, quick release the pressure and remove the lid. Set the corn aside.
- In a blender, add the coconut milk, hemp hearts, nutritional yeast, flour, garlic, cayenne pepper, and salt. Blend until smooth.
- Pour into a saucepan and cook over medium-high heat, stirring constantly. Alternatively, you can add to your Instant Pot and cook at high pressure for 1 minute.
- Stir in the lime juice to the sauce.
- Drizzle the sauce over the corn.
- Serve and enjoy!

Nutrition information per serving:

- Calories: 190
- Fat: 4.6g
- Carbohydrates: 33.6g
- Dietary Fiber: 4.7g
- Protein: 9.3g

6. Great Tasting Sweet Potatoes
Time: 30 minutes
Servings: 4
Freestyle SmartPoints: 5
Ingredients:

- 4 raw sweet potatoes
- 2 cups of water

Instructions:

- Rinse and scrub the sweet potatoes
- Add 2 cups of water and a trivet to your Instant Pot.
- Place the potatoes on top of the trivet.
- Lock the lid and cook at high pressure for 18 minutes.
- When the cooking is done, naturally release the pressure.

- Carefully remove the lid and set the potatoes aside.
- Serve and enjoy!

Nutrition information per serving:

- Calories: 57
- Fat: 1g
- Carbohydrates: 15g
- Dietary Fiber: 2g
- Protein: 1g

7. To-Die-For Brussel Sprouts with Shallots
Time: 15 minutes
Servings: 8
Freestyle SmartPoints: 3
Ingredients:

- 2 pounds of Brussel sprouts, trimmed
- 1 or 2 shallots, finely chopped
- 1 tablespoon of olive oil
- ¼ cup of orange juice
- 2 tablespoons of maple syrup
- 1 teaspoon of salt
- 1 teaspoon of black pepper

Instructions:

- Press "Saute" function on your Instant Pot and add the olive oil.
- Once the oil is hot and ready, add the shallots and cook until brown and crispy, stirring occasionally.
- Turn off "Saute" function on your Instant Pot.
- Add the Brussel sprouts, orange juice, maple syrup, salt, and pepper in your Instant Pot.
- Lock the lid and cook at high pressure for 4 minutes.
- When the cooking is done, quick release the pressure and remove the lid.
- Stir until the Brussel sprouts are covered with the shallots and sauce.
- Serve and enjoy!

Nutrition information per serving:

- Calories: 65
- Fat: 2g
- Carbohydrates: 12g
- Dietary Fiber: 3g
- Protein: 3g

Rice and Grains Recipes
1. Lebanese Hashweh Ground Beef and Rice

Time: 30 minutes
Servings: 6
Freestyle SmartPoints: 5
Ingredients:

- 2 tablespoons of olive oil
- ¼ cup of pine nuts
- 1 cup of onions, sliced
- 1 tablespoon of garlic, minced
- 1 pound of ground beef
- ¼ teaspoon of ground cardamom
- 1 ½ teaspoon of ground allspice
- 1 teaspoon of ground cinnamon
- ¼ teaspoon of ground nutmeg
- 1 cup of basmati rice, rinsed and drained
- 1 teaspoon of salt
- 1 teaspoon of ground black pepper
- 1 cup of water
- ¼ cup of cilantro, chopped

Instructions:

- Press "Sauté" function on your Instant Pot and add the olive oil.
- Once the oil is hot and ready, add the pine nuts and cook for 1 to 2 minutes, stirring frequently.
- Add the minced garlic and onions. Stir well and cook until lightly browned.
- Add the ground beef and cook until brown, breaking up the ground beef with a wooden spoon.

- Add all the spices and stir well.
- Add the rice and 1 cups of water.
- Lock the lid and cook at high pressure for 4 minutes.
- When the cooking is done, naturally release the pressure for 10 minutes and quick release the remaining pressure.
- Fluff the rice with a fork and sprinkle with cilantro. Serve and enjoy!

Nutrition information per serving:

- Calories: 341
- Fat: 13.5g
- Carbohydrates: 27.7g
- Dietary Fiber: 1.1g
- Protein: 26.2g

2. Tastiest Mexican Black Beans and Rice

Time: 30 minutes
Servings: 4
Freestyle SmartPoints: 4
Ingredients:

- 1 (15-ounce) can of black beans, rinsed and drained
- 1 cup of brown rice
- 1 ½ cup of chicken broth
- ¾ cup of picante sauce
- 1 bay leaf
- 1 teaspoon of cumin
- 1 teaspoon of garlic salt
- 1 lime, juice

Toppings:

- Sour cream
- Tortilla chips
- Grated cheese
- Sliced avocados

Instructions:

- Add the black beans, brown rice, chicken broth, picante sauce, bay leaf, cumin, garlic salt, and lime juice to your Instant Pot.
- Lock the lid and cook at high pressure for 22 minutes.
- When the cooking is done, naturally release the pressure for 10 minutes and quick release the remaining pressure.
- Carefully remove the lid and discard the bay leaf.
- Stir the black beans and rice again and add more sauce as needed.
- Ladle into bowls and top with preferred toppings.
- Serve and enjoy!

Nutrition information per serving:

- Calories: 228
- Fat: 1.2g
- Carbohydrates: 44.4g
- Dietary Fiber: 8g
- Protein: 9.9g

3. <u>Kheema Pulao (Indian Meat and Rice)</u>

Time: 30 minutes
Servings: 6
Freestyle SmartPoints: 4
Pulao Ingredients:

- 2 teaspoons of ghee
- 1 red onion, thinly sliced
- 1 tablespoon of ginger, minced
- 1 tablespoon of garlic, minced
- 1 pound of lean ground beef
- 1 ½ teaspoon of salt
- 1 ½ cup of water
- 1 ½ cup of basmati rice
- 1 cup of frozen peas

Spices Ingredients:

- 1 teaspoon of cumin seeds
- 5 whole cloves

- 5 whole peppercorns
- 1 cinnamon stick, broken into pieces
- 3 teaspoons of garam masala

Instructions:

- Press "Saute" function on your Instant Pot and add the ghee.
- Once the ghee is hot, add the spices and cook for 30 seconds, stirring frequently.
- Add the garlic and ginger and cook for 30 seconds, stirring frequently.
- Add the ground beef and cook until lightly brown, stirring frequently and breaking up all the clumps.
- Add the onions, rice, salt, and water and stir until well combined.
- Lock the lid and cook at high pressure for 4 minutes.
- When the cooking is done, naturally release the pressure for 10 minutes and quick release the remaining pressure.
- Remove the lid and stir in the frozen peas.
- Serve and enjoy!

Nutrition information per serving:

- Calories: 354
- Fat: 6.6g
- Carbohydrates: 43.3g
- Dietary Fiber: 2.4g
- Protein: 27.9g

4. Sensational Chicken and Rice
Time: 25 minutes
Servings: 6
Freestyle SmartPoints: 3
Ingredients:

- 1 pound of boneless, skinless chicken thighs
- 1 tablespoon of avocado oil
- 3 small shallots, chopped
- 3 carrots, chopped

- 1 cup of mushrooms, sliced
- 2 garlic cloves, minced
- 1 ½ cup of white jasmine rice, rinsed and drained
- 1 ½ cup of chicken stock
- 2 tablespoons of fresh thyme leaves, chopped
- 1 teaspoon of salt
- 1 teaspoon of black pepper

Instructions:

- Press "Saute" function on your Instant Pot and add the avocado oil.
- Season the chicken thighs with salt and pepper.
- Once the oil is hot, add the chicken thighs and cook for 5 minutes per side.
- Remove the chicken and set aside.
- Add 1/3 cup of chicken stock to deglaze your Instant Pot. Scrape the bits with a wooden spoon.
- Add the shallots, mushroom, and carrots, and cook for 3 minutes, stirring frequently.
- Add the garlic and cook for 1 minute, stirring frequently.
- Add the chicken stock, rice, thyme and stir until well combined.
- Place the chicken thighs on top of the mixture.
- Lock the lid and cook at high pressure for 10 minutes.
- When the cooking is done, naturally release the pressure and remove the lid.
- Remove the chicken and shred using 2 forks.
- Return the chicken to your Instant Pot and stir.
- Serve and enjoy!

Nutrition information per serving:

- Calories: 347
- Fat: 6.5g
- Carbohydrates: 43.8g
- Dietary Fiber: 1.9g
- Protein: 26.5g

5. Scrumptious Mexican Rice

Time: 18 minutes
Servings: 12
Freestyle SmartPoints: 4
Ingredients:

- 2 tablespoons of avocado oil
- ¼ cup of onions, chopped
- 4 garlic cloves, minced
- 2 cusp of white rice
- 1 teaspoon of salt
- ¾ cups of crushed tomatoes
- 2 ½ cups of chicken stock
- ½ teaspoon of cumin
- ½ teaspoon of garlic powder
- ½ teaspoon of smoked paprika
- ¼ cup of cilantro, chopped

Instructions:

- Press "Saute" function on your Instant Pot and add the avocado oil.
- Once the oil is hot, add the onions and garlic. Cook for 3 minutes or until browned, stirring occasionally.
- Add the white rice and stir the rice until well coated with the oil, garlic, and onions.
- Add the chicken stock, crushed tomatoes, cilantro, cumin, smoked paprika, garlic powder, and salt.
- Lock the lid and cook at high pressure for 8 minutes.
- When the cooking is done, naturally release the pressure for5 minutes and quick release the remaining pressure.
- Remove the lid. Take a fork and lightly fluff the rice through.
- Serve and enjoy!

Nutrition information per serving:

- Calories: 510
- Fat: 14.2g
- Carbohydrates: 80.3g

- Dietary Fiber: 2.9g
- Protein: 13.6g

Soups, Stews, and Broths Recipes
1. Lovely Curry Cauliflower and Broccoli Soup
Time: 30 minutes
Servings: 8
Freestyle SmartPoints: 3
Ingredients:

- 1 large cauliflower head, chopped
- 1 large broccoli head, chopped
- 1 red bell pepper, chopped
- 1 green bell pepper, chopped
- 4 sweet potatoes, chopped
- 1 onion, finely chopped
- 2 garlic cloves, minced
- 2 cups of unsweetened coconut milk
- 2 cups of vegetable broth
- 1 tablespoon of coconut oil
- 2 tablespoons of yellow curry powder
- 1 teaspoon of cumin
- 1 teaspoon of dried thyme
- ½ teaspoon of cayenne pepper
- 1 teaspoon of salt
- 1 teaspoon of black pepper

Instructions:

- Press "saute" setting on your Instant Pot and add the coconut oil.
- Once the oil is hot and ready, add the onions and cook until translucent, stirring frequently.
- Add the garlic and cook for 1 minute or until fragrant.
- Add the cauliflower, broccoli, and red bell pepper. Cook for an additional minute, stirring occasionally.
- Add the remaining ingredients except for the coconut milk in your Instant Pot.
- Close the lid and cook at high pressure for 3 minutes.

- When the cooking is done, quick release the pressure and remove the lid.
- Stir in the coconut milk and adjust the seasoning as needed. Serve and enjoy!

Nutrition information per serving:

- Calories: 264
- Fat: 16.7g
- Carbohydrates: 26.4g
- Dietary Fiber: 7.2g
- Protein: 6.5g

2. **Flavorful Chicken Tortilla-Less Soup**

Time: 30 minutes
Servings: 8
Freestyle SmartPoints: 2
Ingredients:

- 1 ½ pounds of boneless, skinless chicken breasts
- 2 (10-ounce) cans of diced tomatoes and green chilies
- 1 (14.5-ounce) cans of chicken broth
- 2 zucchinis, chopped
- 1 ¾ cups of low-fat coconut cream
- 2 chipotle peppers in adobo sauce
- 2 teaspoons of adobo sauce
- 1 medium onion, chopped
- 2 teaspoons of garlic powder
- 1 teaspoon of onion powder
- 1 teaspoon of cumin
- 2 teaspoon of chili powder
- 1 teaspoon of dried oregano
- 1 teaspoon of smoked paprika
- 1 teaspoon of salt

Instructions:

- Add all the ingredients except for the coconut cream into your Instant Pot.

- Close and seal the lid.
- Cook at high pressure for 20 minutes.
- When the cooking is done, naturally release the pressure for 10 minutes and quick release any remaining pressure.
- Remove the chicken and chop into pieces.
- Return the cubed chicken to your Instant Pot and stir in the coconut cream.
- Serve and enjoy!

Nutrition information per serving:

- Calories: 169
- Fat: 3.1g
- Carbohydrates: 7.4g
- Dietary Fiber: 1.9g
- Protein: 27.3g

3. Curried Carrot Red Lentil Soup

Time: 35 minutes
Servings: 4
Freestyle SmartPoints: 3
Ingredients:

- 2 teaspoons of olive oil
- 1 cup of onions, chopped
- 1 tablespoon of ginger, grated
- 1 tablespoon of curry powder
- 2 cups of baby carrots, peeled and diced
- 4 cups of vegetable broth
- ¾ cups of dried red lentils rinsed well
- 1 teaspoons of salt
- ¼ teaspoon of ground black pepper

Instructions:

- Press "saute" function on your Instant Pot and add the olive oil.
- Once the oil is hot and ready, add the onions and cook until translucent, stirring frequently.

- Add the ginger and curry powder and cook for 30 seconds, stirring frequently.
- Add the carrots, vegetable broth, red lentils, salt, and black pepper. Stir until well combined.
- Lock the lid and cook at high pressure for 10 minutes.
- When the cooking is done, quick release the pressure and remove the lid.
- Use an immersion blender to puree the soup until smooth.
- Adjust the seasoning as needed.
- Serve and enjoy!

Nutrition information per serving:

- Calories: 209
- Fat: 4.4g
- Carbohydrates: 27.7g
- Dietary Fiber: 12.5g
- Protein: 14.8g

4.   Scrumptious Sausage Italian Lentil and Barley Soup

Time: 25 minutes
Servings: 12
Freestyle SmartPoints: 2
Ingredients:

- 2 tablespoons of olive oil
- 1 pound of Italian sausage
- 1 ½ cup of dry lentils, rinsed
- 1 cup of kale, stemmed and finely chopped
- 1/3 cup of pearl barley
- 4 carrots, peeled and chopped
- 1 tablespoon of tomato paste
- 2 celery stalks, chopped
- 1 cup of onions, chopped
- 2 garlic cloves, minced
- 1 tablespoon of Italian seasoning
- ¼ teaspoon of red pepper flakes
- 1 teaspoon of salt
- 1 teaspoon of black pepper

- 5 cups of chicken stock
- 2 (15-ounce) can of crushed tomatoes
- ¼ cup of parsley, chopped
- 2 tablespoons of cider vinegar

Instructions:

- Press "saute" function on your Instant Pot and add the olive oil.
- Once the oil is hot and ready, add the Italian sausage and cook until no longer pink, breaking into smaller pieces with a spoon as you cook.
- Add the onions, celery, and carrots. Cook for 3 to 4 minutes or until the vegetables has softened.
- Stir in the garlic, tomato paste, Italian seasoning, parsley, red pepper flakes, and salt.
- Add the diced tomatoes, cider vinegar, pearl barley, beef stock, and lentils. Stir until well combined.
- Close the lid and cook at high pressure for 10 minutes.
- When the cooking is done, naturally release the pressure for 10 minutes and quick release any remaining pressure.
- Remove the lid and stir in the kale. Serve and enjoy!

Nutrition information per serving:

- Calories: 303
- Fat: 13.6g
- Carbohydrates: 28.8g
- Dietary Fiber: 11.4g
- Protein: 16.7g

5. Delectable Curry Pumpkin

Time: 20 minutes
Servings: 6
Freestyle SmartPoints: 4
Ingredients:

- 1 onion, chopped
- 2 teaspoons of olive oil
- 2 tablespoons of butter

- 3 tablespoons of all-purpose flour
- 2 tablespoons of curry powder
- 5 cups of vegetable broth
- 4 cups of pumpkin puree
- 1 ½ cups of low-fat coconut cream
- 2 tablespoons of soy sauce
- ½ tablespoon of brown sugar
- 1 teaspoon of lemon juice
- ½ teaspoon of lemon zest
- ¼ teaspoon of cayenne pepper
- ½ teaspoon of salt
- ½ teaspoon of black pepper

Instructions:

- Press "saute" function on your Instant Pot and add the olive oil.
- When the oil is hot and ready, add the onions and cook until softened.
- Remove and set aside.
- Melt the butter in your Instant Pot and stir in the flour and curry powder until smooth.
- Continue to stir until the mixture begins to bubble.
- Gradually stir in the vegetable broth.
- Add the pumpkin, onions, soy sauce, brown sugar, salt, and black pepper into your Instant Pot.
- Close the lid and cook at high pressure for 3 minutes.
- When the cooking is done, quick release the pressure and remove the lid.
- Stir in the coconut cream.
- Use an immersion blender and blend until smooth.
- Stir in the lemon juice and lemon zest. Serve and enjoy!

Nutrition information per serving:

- Calories: 307
- Fat: 21.7g
- Carbohydrates: 24.4g
- Dietary Fiber: 7.3g
- Protein: 8.5g

6. Hearty Golden Lentil and Spinach Soup

Time: 35 minutes
Servings: 4
Freestyle SmartPoints:
Ingredients:

- 2 teaspoons of olive oil
- 1 cup of onions, chopped
- 1 cup of carrots, chopped
- ½ cup of celery, chopped
- 4 garlic cloves, minced
- 2 teaspoons of ground cumin
- 1 teaspoon of ground turmeric
- 1 teaspoon of dried thyme
- 1 teaspoon of salt
- ¼ teaspoon of black pepper
- 1 cup of dry brown lentils, rinsed
- 4 cups of vegetable broth
- 6 cups of baby spinach

Instructions:

- Press "saute" function on your Instant Pot and add the olive oil.
- When the oil is hot and ready, add the onions, carrots, and celery. Cook until tender, stirring occasionally.
- Add the garlic, cumin, turmeric, thyme, salt, and black pepper. Cook for 1 minute, stirring constantly.
- Add the lentils and pour in the vegetable broth. Stir until well combined.
- Lock the lid on your Instant Pot and cook at high pressure for 12 minutes.
- When the cooking is done, quick release the pressure and remove the lid.
- Stir in the spinach until wilted.
- Serve and enjoy!

Nutrition information per serving:

- Calories: 98

- Fat: 4g
- Carbohydrates: 9.3g
- Dietary Fiber: 2.6g
- Protein: 7g

7. **Delicious Italian Farmhouse Vegetable Soup**

Time: 25 minutes
Servings: 4
Freestyle SmartPoints: 0
Ingredients:

- 1 tablespoon of olive oil
- 1 onion, chopped
- 2 celery sticks, sliced
- 2 carrots, peeled and sliced
- 6 mushrooms, sliced
- 4 porcini mushrooms, sliced
- 4 garlic cloves, minced
- ½ long red chili, sliced
- 2 cups of kale, stemmed and chopped
- 1 zucchini, chopped
- 1 cup of tomatoes, chopped
- 4 cups of vegetable stock
- 1 tablespoon of lemon juice
- 1 teaspoon of lemon zest
- 1 teaspoon of salt
- 1 teaspoon of black pepper

Instructions:

- Press "saute" function on your Instant Pot and add the olive oil.
- Once the oil is hot and ready, add the onion, salt, celery, and carrots. Cook for 2 minutes, stirring occasionally.
- Add the mushrooms, chili, and garlic. Cook for 1 minute, stirring occasionally.
- Add the remaining ingredients and stir until well combined.
- Lock the lid and cook at high pressure for 10 minutes.
- When the cooking is done, naturally release the pressure for 10

minutes and quick release any remaining pressure. Carefully remove the lid.
- Serve and enjoy!

Nutrition information per serving:

- Calories: 106
- Fat: 4.4g
- Carbohydrates: 15.1g
- Dietary Fiber: 3.3g
- Protein: 4.1g

8. Creamy Cauliflower Soup
Time: 30 minutes
Servings: 5
Freestyle SmartPoints: 2
Ingredients:

- 2 tablespoons of olive oil
- 1 onion, chopped
- 2 garlic cloves, minced
- 2 carrots, shredded
- 1 large head of cauliflower, chopped
- 1 cup of coconut cream
- 2/3 cup of mozzarella cheese, grated
- 1/3 cup of parmesan cheese, grated
- 2 cups of vegetable broth
- ¼ cup of butter
- ¼ cup of all-purpose flour
- 1 tablespoon of parsley
- 1 teaspoon of salt
- 1 teaspoon of black pepper

Instructions:

- Press "saute" setting on your Instant Pot and add the butter.
- Once the butter has melted, add the onions and cook until tender and golden.
- Add the garlic and cook for 1 minute.

- Add the carrots, cauliflower, vegetable broth, salt, and black pepper.
- Close the lid and cook at high pressure for 5 minutes.
- When the cooking is done, naturally release the pressure for 5 minutes and quick release any remaining pressure.
- Remove the lid from your Instant Pot.
- In a saucepan over medium-high heat, melt ¼ cup of butter.
- Stir in the ¼ cup of flour and stir until the mixture thickens and turns golden brown.
- Add the mozzarella cheese, parmesan cheese, and coconut cream in your Instant Pot and stir until melted.
- Add the flour mixture to the soup and stir until thickened.
- Garnish with parsley and adjust the seasoning as needed. Serve and enjoy!

Nutrition information per serving:

- Calories: 405
- Fat: 31.3g
- Carbohydrates: 22.3g
- Dietary Fiber: 6.6g
- Protein: 14.1g

9. Supreme Taco Soup

Time: 30 minutes
Servings: 10
Freestyle SmartPoints: 0
Ingredients:

- 1 ½ pound of ground turkey breast
- 1 large onion, chopped
- 1 tablespoon of olive oil
- 2 tablespoons of package Hidden Valley ranch dressing
- 2 tablespoons of taco seasoning mix
- 4 cups of chicken broth
- 1 (15-ounce) can of pinto beans
- 1 (15-ounce) can of hot chili beans
- 1 (15-ounce) can of whole kernel corns
- 1 (15-ounce) can of stewed tomatoes, Mexican flavor

- 1 (15-ounce) can of stewed tomatoes, any flavor
- 1 teaspoon of garlic powder
- 1 teaspoon of salt
- 1 teaspoon of black pepper

Instructions:

- Press "saute" function on your Instant Pot and add the ground turkey.
- Cook until the turkey is browned, stirring frequently.
- Add the olive oil and onions and cook for 5 minutes or until onions have softened.
- Add the remaining ingredients to your Instant Pot.
- Lock the lid and cook at high pressure for 15 minutes.
- When the cooking is done, quick release the pressure and remove the lid.
- Stir the soup again and adjust the seasoning as needed.
- Serve and enjoy!

Nutrition information per serving:

- Calories: 249
- Fat: 3g
- Carbohydrates: 39g
- Dietary Fiber: 8g
- Protein: 19g

10. **Yummy Tomato Spinach Soup**
Time: 20 minutes
Servings: 6
Freestyle SmartPoints: 1
Ingredients:

- 1 onion, chopped
- 2 garlic cloves, minced
- 2 carrots, grated
- 2 tablespoons of olive oil
- 1 pound of fresh spinach
- 1 (28-ounce) can of crushed tomatoes

- 1 ½ cups of chicken broth
- 2 teaspoons of dried basil
- 1 teaspoon of salt
- 1 teaspoon of black pepper
- 1 (5-ounce) can of evaporated milk

Instructions:

- Press "saute" setting on your Instant Pot and add the olive oil.
- Once the oil is hot, add the onions and carrots and cook until softened, stirring occasionally.
- Add the garlic and cook for 1 minute or until fragrant.
- Add the remaining ingredients except for the spinach and evaporated milk.
- Lock the lid and cook at high pressure for 15 minutes.
- When the cooking is done, naturally release the pressure for 10 minutes and quick release any remaining pressure.
- Remove the lid and carefully stir in the evaporated milk and spinach.
- Serve and enjoy!

Nutrition information per serving:

- Calories: 169
- Fat: 7.1g
- Carbohydrates: 20g
- Dietary Fiber: 6.8g
- Protein: 8.6g

11. Flavorsome Chunky Beef, Cabbage, and Tomato Soup
Time: 30 minutes
Servings: 7
Freestyle SmartPoints: 3
Ingredients:

- 1 pound of ground beef
- 1 onion, chopped
- 2 celery stalks, chopped
- 2 carrots, chopped

- 1 (28-ounce) can of diced tomatoes
- 5 cups of green cabbage, chopped
- 4 cups of beef stock
- 2 bay leaves
- 1 teaspoon of garlic powder
- 1 teaspoon of salt
- 1 teaspoon of black pepper

Instructions:

- Press "saute" function on your Instant Pot and add the olive oil.
- When the oil is hot, add the ground beef and cook until brown.
- When the ground beef has browned, add the onions, celery, and carrots and cook for 4 minutes or until softened.
- Add the tomatoes, cabbage, beef stock, and bay leaves.
- Lock the lid and cook at high pressure for 20 minutes.
- When the cooking is done, naturally release the pressure and remove the lid.
- Remove the bay leaves.
- Serve and enjoy!

Nutrition information per serving:

- Calories: 181
- Fat: 6g
- Carbohydrates: 14g
- Dietary Fiber: 2g
- Protein: 15.5g

12. Unique Loaded Baked Potato Soup

Time: 25 minutes
Servings: 6
Freestyle SmartPoints: 7
Ingredients:

- 2 pounds of potatoes
- 5 bacon slices, chopped
- ¼ cup of butter
- ¼ cup of flour

- 4 cups of milk
- ½ cup of sour cream
- ½ cup of cheddar cheese, grated
- 3 green onions, diced
- 1 teaspoon of bouillon chicken base
- 1 teaspoon of salt
- ½ teaspoon of black pepper

Instructions:

- Press "saute" function on your Instant Pot and add the bacon bits.
- Cook the bacon until brown and crispy. Once done, remove the bacon and set aside. Turn off "saute" function.
- Add 1 cup of water and a trivet inside your Instant Pot.
- Place the potatoes on top of the trivet.
- Lock the lid and cook at high pressure for 10 minutes.
- When the cooking is done, quick release the pressure and remove the lid.
- Remove the potatoes and set aside.
- Remove the water and discard the trivet.
- Press "saute" setting on your Instant Pot and add the butter.
- Once the butter has melted, add 1 tablespoon of flour and stir until begins to bubble. Add the milk and bouillon and start to whisk.
- Stir in the sour cream, cheddar cheese, diced onions, and bacon.
- Smash the potatoes with a potato masher and stir the potatoes into the soup.
- Add salt and black pepper to the soup. Serve and enjoy!

Nutrition information per serving:

- Calories: 439
- Fat: 25g
- Carbohydrates: 37.5g
- Dietary Fiber: 4g
- Protein: 17.5g

13. <u>Exquisite Broccoli Cheese Soup</u>

Time: 15 minutes
Servings: 6
Freestyle SmartPoints: 2
Ingredients:

- ¼ cup of butter
- 1 onion, finely chopped
- 2 cups of carrots, chopped
- 2 garlic cloves, minced
- ¼ cup of flour
- 3 cups of vegetable stock
- 6 cups of broccoli florets
- 1 teaspoon of paprika
- 1 teaspoon of Dijon mustard
- 1 ½ cups of Monterey jack cheese, shredded
- 1 ½ cups of sharp cheddar cheese, shredded
- ½ cup of milk
- ½ cup of coconut cream
- 1 teaspoon of salt
- 1 teaspoon of black pepper

Instructions:

- Press "saute" setting on your Instant Pot and add the butter.
- When the butter is melted, add the onions and carrots and cook for 3 minutes or until onions are translucent.
- Stir in the garlic and flour and cook for 1 minute.
- Stir in the broth and continue to stir until flour lumps are gone.
- Add the broccoli and vegetable stock to your Instant Pot.
- Lock the lid and cook at high pressure for 8 minutes.
- When the cooking is done, quick release the pressure and remove the lid.
- Stir in the paprika, Dijon mustard, salt, and black pepper until well incorporated.
- Stir in the cheeses until fully melted.
- Once the cheese has melted, add the milk and coconut cream.
- If you prefer, use an immersion blender to blend the soup until reached your desired consistency. Serve and enjoy!

Nutrition information per serving:

- Calories: 228
- Fat: 14.6g
- Carbohydrates: 18.5g
- Dietary Fiber: 5.1g
- Protein: 7.2g

Appetizers and Side Dishes Recipes
1. Cheesy Rotel Queso Dip
Time: 20 minutes
Servings: 11
Freestyle SmartPoints: 2
Ingredients:

- 2 cups of ground Italian sausage
- 1 (10-ounce) can of Rotel tomatoes with chiles, diced and drained
- 2 jalapenos, seeded and diced
- 1 poblano pepper, diced
- 1 cup of onions, minced
- 3 garlic cloves, minced
- 2 teaspoons of canola oil
- ¼ cup of cilantro, chopped
- 2 cups of shredded reduced-fat sharp Cheddar, Sargento
- ½ cup of low sodium chicken broth
- 1 cup of skim milk
- 3 tablespoons of cornstarch
- 1 lime, juice and zest
- ½ teaspoon of ground cumin
- 1 teaspoon of ancho chili powder

Instructions:

- In a small bowl, mix ¼ cup of skim milk with 3 tablespoons of cornstarch. Set aside. Press "saute" function on your Instant Pot and add the canola oil.
- Once the oil is hot and ready, add the onions, garlic, poblano, and jalapeno. Cook until softened, about 5 to 7 minutes, stirring

frequently.

- Turn off "saute" function on your Instant Pot.
- Add the chicken broth, sausage, tomatoes, and 1 cup of cheese to your Instant Pot. Lock the lid and cook at high pressure for 5 minutes.
- When the cooking is done, naturally release the pressure for 5 minutes and quick release the remaining pressure.
- Press "saute" function on your Instant Pot and stir in the remaining ingredients.
- Cook and stir until the cheese has completely melted. Serve and enjoy!

Nutrition information per serving:

- Calories: 92.5
- Fat: 4.6g
- Carbohydrates: 7g
- Dietary Fiber: 1g
- Protein: 6.5g

2. Cabbage with Turkey Sausage

Time: 10 minutes
Servings: 8
Freestyle SmartPoints: 2
Ingredients:

- 1 pound of Turkey sausage, sliced
- 1 large cabbage head, chopped
- 1 onion, chopped
- 3 garlic cloves, minced
- 2 teaspoons of sugar
- 2 teaspoons of balsamic vinegar
- 2 teaspoons of Dijon mustard
- 1 tablespoon of olive oil
- 1 teaspoon of salt
- 1 teaspoon of black pepper

Instructions:

- Press "Saute" function on your Instant Pot and add the olive oil.
- Once the oil is hot and ready, add the Turkey sausage and onions. Cook until slightly browned.
- Add the cabbage and remaining ingredients to your Instant Pot. Cook until the cabbage cooks down, stirring frequently.
- Turn off "Saute" function on your Instant Pot. Adjust the seasoning as needed.
- Serve and enjoy!

Nutrition information per serving:

- Calories: 220
- Fat: 17.9g
- Carbohydrates: 3g
- Dietary Fiber: 0.5g
- Protein: 11.3g

3.   Fit for a King Spinach Artichoke Macaroni and Cheese

Time: 25 minutes
Servings: 6
Freestyle SmartPoints: 6
Ingredients:

- 2 tablespoons of olive oil
- 1 large onion, finely chopped
- 10 garlic cloves, minced
- 1 can of artichoke hearts, drained and roughly chopped
- 1 pound of pasta
- 12-ounces of baby spinach
- 6 cups of vegetable broth
- 1 teaspoon of red pepper flakes
- 1 teaspoon of salt
- 1 teaspoon of black pepper
- 4-ounces of cream cheese softened
- ¼ cup of parmesan cheese, grated
- 1 cup of shredded low-fat mozzarella

Instructions:

- Press "saute" function on your Instant Pot and add the olive oil.
- Once the oil is hot and ready, add the onions and cook for 2 minutes or until translucent.
- Add the garlic and cook for 1 minute or until fragrant, stirring frequently.
- Add the artichoke hearts and cook for another minute.
- Add the pasta and 5 cups of vegetable broth.
- Lock the lid and cook at high pressure for 4 minutes.
- When the cooking is done, quick release the pressure and remove the lid.
- Stir in the remaining vegetable broth. If the pasta looks watery, don't add.
- Press "saute" function on your Instant Pot and fold in the baby spinach. Cook until the spinach wilts.
- Stir in the cream cheese, mozzarella, and parmesan.
- Season with red pepper flakes, salt, and black pepper. Stir everything until everything is well combined and the cheese has melted. Serve and enjoy!

Nutrition information per serving:

- Calories: 509
- Fat: 18g
- Carbohydrates: 65g
- Dietary Fiber: 4g
- Protein: 22g

4. **Smoky Baked Beans**
Time: 45 minutes
Servings: 12
Freestyle SmartPoints: 2
Ingredients:

- 1 pound of dried navy beans, soaked overnight and rinsed
- 1 tablespoon of salt
- 8 slices of bacon, cut into ½-inch pieces
- 1 large onion, chopped
- 2 ½ cups of chicken stock
- ½ cup of molasses

- ½ cup of ketchup
- ¼ cup of packed brown sugar
- 1 teaspoon of dry mustard
- ½ teaspoon of black pepper

Instructions:

- Press "saute" function on your Instant Pot and add the bacon bits. Cook until brown and crispy, stirring occasionally.
- Remove the bacon bits and place on paper towels.
- Add the onions to the bacon grease and cook until tender, about 3 minutes.
- Add the chicken stock, molasses, ketchup, brown sugar, dry mustard, salt, and black pepper to your Instant Pot. Stir until well combined.
- Stir in the soaked navy beans.
- Lock the lid and cook at high pressure for 35 minutes.
- When the cooking is done, naturally release the pressure for 10 minutes and quick release any remaining pressure. Remove the lid.
- Stir in the cooked bacon and press "saute" function. Simmer the beans, stirring occasionally, until the sauce reaches your desired consistency.
- Serve and enjoy!

Nutrition information per serving:

- Calories: 264
- Fat: 6.1g
- Carbohydrates: 40g
- Dietary Fiber: 9.5g
- Protein: 13.6g

5.   Classic Potato Salad
Time: 10 minutes + 1 hour of refrigerating time
Servings: 8
Freestyle SmartPoints: 3
Ingredients:

- 6 medium russet potatoes, peeled and cubed
- 1 ½ cup of water
- 4 large eggs
- ¼ cup of onions, finely chopped
- 1 cup of fat-free mayonnaise
- 2 tablespoons of parsley
- 1 tablespoon of pickle juice
- 1 tablespoon of mustard
- ½ teaspoon of salt
- ½ teaspoon of black pepper

Instructions:

- Place a steamer basket inside your Instant Pot.
- Add the water, potatoes, and eggs.
- Lock the lid and cook at high pressure for 4 minutes.
- When the cooking is done, quick release the pressure and remove the lid.
- Remove the steamer basket from your Instant Pot and place the eggs in an ice bath.
- Allow the potatoes to cool. Peel and dice the cooled eggs.
- In a large bowl, combine the onions, mayonnaise, pickle juice, and mustard.
- Stir in the potatoes and eggs into the potato salad.
- Season with salt and black pepper. Refrigerate for 1 hour before serving.

Nutrition information per serving:

- Calories: 258
- Fat: 12.2g
- Carbohydrates: 32.7g
- Dietary Fiber: 3.9g
- Protein: 5.8g

6. Contest-Winning Chili Con Carne
Time: 20 minutes
Servings: 8
Freestyle SmartPoints: 8

Ingredients:

- 1 pound of ground beef
- 1 (28-ounce) can of whole peeled tomatoes, undrained
- 1 (14-ounce) can of black beans, rinsed and drained
- 1 (14-ounce) can of kidney beans, rinsed and drained
- 3 tablespoons of olive oil
- 1 large onion, finely chopped
- 1 red bell pepper, chopped
- 2 medium jalapenos, chopped
- 2 garlic cloves, minced
- 1 teaspoon of ground cumin
- 1 tablespoon of chili powder
- 1 teaspoon of dried oregano
- 1 ½ teaspoon of salt
- ½ teaspoon of black pepper

Instructions:

- Press "saute" function on your Instant Pot and add the olive oil.
- Once the oil is hot and ready, add the ground beef and cook until brown, breaking it into smaller pieces with a spoon.
- Add the onions, bell pepper, and jalapenos into your Instant Pot and cook for 3 minutes.
- Add the garlic, cumin, chili powder, oregano, salt, and black pepper. Cook for 1 minute, stirring occasionally.
- Add the Worcestershire sauce, tomatoes, water, and beans. Stir until well combined.
- Lock the lid on your Instant Pot and cook at high pressure for 10 minutes.
- When the cooking is done, naturally release the pressure for 10 minutes and quick release any remaining pressure.
- Press "saute" function and cook until the chili has thickened or reached your desired consistency. Serve and enjoy!

Nutrition information per serving:

- Calories: 519
- Fat: 10.3g

- Carbohydrates: 68.6g
- Dietary Fiber: 17g
- Protein: 40.4g

7. Drive-Thru Tacos

Time: 20 minutes
Servings: 4
Freestyle SmartPoints: 6
Ingredients:

- 1 pound of ground beef
- 1 tablespoon of Worcestershire sauce
- 1 tablespoon of olive oil
- 1 cup of beef broth
- 2 teaspoons of all-purpose flour
- 1 tablespoon of chili powder
- ¼ teaspoon of garlic powder
- ¼ teaspoon of onion powder
- ¼ teaspoon of dried minced onions
- 1 ½ teaspoon of ground cumin
- ¼ teaspoon of dried oregano
- ½ teaspoon of paprika
- 1 teaspoon of salt
- ½ teaspoon of black pepper
- A pinch of cayenne pepper
- Taco shells (for serving)

Instructions:

- Press "saute" function on your Instant Pot and add the olive oil.
- Once hot and ready, add the ground beef and cook until brown, stirring occasionally.
- Turn off "saute" function.
- Add the remaining ingredients in your Instant Pot. Stir until well combined.
- Lock the lid and cook at high pressure for 3 minutes.
- When the cooking is done, naturally release the pressure for 10 minutes and quick release any remaining pressure.

- Remove the lid and press "saute" function. Mix and allow to simmer until most of the liquid has reduced.
- Spoon the taco meat onto taco shells.
- Serve and enjoy!

Nutrition information per serving:

- Calories: 259
- Fat: 10.9g
- Carbohydrates: 2g
- Dietary Fiber: 0g
- Protein: 35.7g

8.   Fun to Eat Monkey Bread

Time: 25 minutes
Servings: 8
Freestyle SmartPoints: 5
Ingredients:

- 3 ½ cups of all-purpose flour
- ¾ cups of sugar
- ¼-ounces of active dry variety yeast
- 1 teaspoon of salt
- 1 cup of low-fat milk
- ½ cup of unsalted butter softened
- 1 large egg, beaten
- 1 teaspoon of ground cinnamon
- ¼ teaspoon of ground nutmeg
- 1/8 teaspoon of cloves

Instructions:

- In a large bowl, add 1 ½ cup of all-purpose flour, ¼ cup of sugar, yeast, and salt. Mix well.
- Use an electric mixer and gradually beat in the milk and ¼ cup of butter.
- Add the egg and remaining flour and beat for 2 minutes.
- Turn the dough onto a floured counter and knead until smooth and elastic.

- Cover the dough with plastic wrap and allow to rest for 10 minutes.
- In a small bowl, add ¼ cup of melted butter.
- In a second bowl, add ½ cup of sugar, cinnamon, nutmeg, and cloves.
- Divide the dough into 4 quarters.
- Dip each dough quarter into the butter mixture and coat well with the sugar mixture.
- Place the biscuit pieces into a greased mini loaf pan.
- Add 1 cup of water and a trivet to your Instant Pot.
- Place the loaf pan on top of the trivet. Cover with a piece of aluminum foil.
- Lock the lid and cook at high pressure for 21 minutes.
- When the cooking is done, naturally release the pressure for 5 minutes and quick release any remaining pressure.
- Remove the lid and allow the bread to cool Serve and enjoy!

Nutrition information per serving:

- Calories: 398
- Fat: 13.3g
- Carbohydrates: 62.4g
- Dietary Fiber: 1.7g
- Protein: 7.9g

9. Perfect Little Smokies
Time: 10 minutes
Servings: 8
Freestyle SmartPoints: 2
Ingredients:

- 2 (12-ounce) packages of Cocktail Sausages
- 8-ounces of barbecue sauce
- ¼ cup of light brown sugar
- 1 tablespoon of white vinegar
- 1 tablespoon of honey
- 4-ounces of beer

Instructions:

- Add the sausages to your Instant Pot.
- Add the barbecue sauce, brown sugar, white vinegar, honey, and beer to the sausages. Stir until well combined.
- Lock the lid and cook at high pressure for 1minute.
- When the cooking is done, naturally release the pressure for 1 minute and quick release the remaining pressure.
- Press "Saute" in your Instant Pot. Cook and stir for 5 minutes to thicken the sauce.
- Serve and enjoy!

Nutrition information per serving:

- Calories: 363
- Fat: 24.2g
- Carbohydrates: 17.4g
- Dietary Fiber: 0.2g
- Protein: 16.6g

Desserts Recipes
1.   Secret Chocolate Cupcakes
Time: 40 minutes
Servings: 8
Freestyle SmartPoints: 4
Cupcake Ingredients:

- 1 box of chocolate cake mix
- 1 (15-ounce) can of pumpkin
- ¼ cup of water

Frosting ingredients:

- ¼ cup of peanut butter
- 1 teaspoons of cocoa powder
- 2 tablespoons of maple syrup

Instructions:

- In a large bowl, add and mix all the cupcake ingredients.
- Fill silicone cupcake liners ¾ full. If you don't have silicone

cupcake liners, you can use ramekins or heat-safe glass jars. Cover with aluminum foil.
- Add 1 ½ cups of water and a trivet inside your Instant Pot.
- Place the cupcakes on the trivet.
- Close the lid and cook at high pressure for 25 minutes.
- When the cooking is done, naturally release the pressure and remove the lid.
- Carefully remove the cupcakes and allow to cool.
- In a bowl, add and mix all the frosting ingredients until well combined.
- Spoon the frosting on top of the cupcakes.
- Serve and enjoy

Nutrition information per serving:

- Calories: 359
- Fat: 14.5g
- Carbohydrates: 57.2g
- Dietary Fiber: 3.7g
- Protein: 6.5g

2. Satisfying Blueberry Compote

Time: 20 minutes
Servings: 2
Freestyle SmartPoints: 4
Ingredients:

- 3 cups of frozen blueberries
- ¾ cups of sugar
- 2 tablespoons of lemon juice
- 2 tablespoons of cornstarch
- 2 tablespoons of water

Instructions:

- Add the blueberries, sugar, and lemon juice inside your Instant Pot. Stir until well combined.
- Lock the lid and cook at high pressure for 3 minutes.

- When the cooking is done, naturally release the pressure for 10 minutes and quick release any remaining pressure.
- In a small bowl, mix the cornstarch with the water.
- Press saute on your Instant Pot and stir in the cornstarch mixture until thickened.
- Place in a storage container and refrigerate for at least 3 hours.
- Serve and enjoy!

Nutrition information per serving:

- Calories: 440
- Fat: 0.9g
- Carbohydrates: 114.1g
- Dietary Fiber: 5.4g
- Protein: 1.9g

3. **Elegant Blackberry Cobbler**
Time: 20 minutes
Servings: 6
Freestyle SmartPoints: 6
Ingredients:

- 1 (12-ounce) package of fresh blackberries, washed and dry
- 8-ounces of white cake mix
- ¼ cup of butter
- 1 cup of water

Instructions:

- Grease an oven safe dish that will fit in your Instant Pot with nonstick cooking spray.
- Add the blackberries to the dish.
- In a bowl, using a pastry blender cut the butter into the cake mix until resembles crumbly texture.
- Spread the cake mixture over the blackberries.
- Tightly cover with aluminum foil.
- Add 1 cup of water and a trivet inside your Instant Pot.
- Place the oven safe dish on top.

- Lock the lid of your Instant Pot and cook at high pressure for 10 minutes.
- When the cooking is done, naturally release the pressure for 10 minutes and quick release any remaining pressure.
- Remove the lid and carefully remove the dish from your Instant Pot.
- Allow cooling for 10 minutes.
- Serve and enjoy!

Nutrition information per serving:

- Calories: 253
- Fat: 12.1g
- Carbohydrates: 34.9g
- Dietary Fiber: 3.4g
- Protein: 2.6g

4. Glorious Chocolate Chip Bundt Cake

Time: 40 minutes
Servings: 12
Freestyle SmartPoints: 6
Ingredients:

- 1 (16.5-ounces) of chocolate fudge cake mix
- 2 tablespoons of all-purpose flour
- 1 (3-ounce) package of chocolate dry pudding mix
- 1 cup of buttermilk
- ½ cup of warm water
- ¼ cup of unsweetened applesauce
- 2 tablespoons of coconut oil
- 1 teaspoon of vanilla extract
- 2 large eggs, beaten
- 1 cup of chocolate chips

Topping ingredients:

- 2 tablespoons of powdered sugar

Instructions:

- In a large bowl, add all the cake ingredients except for the chocolate chips and mix until well combined.
- Fold in the chocolate chips.
- Grease a bundt pan with nonstick cooking spray.
- Pour the cake batter into the greased bundt pan.
- Tightly cover the bundt pan with aluminum foil.
- Add 1 ½ cups of water and a trivet inside your Instant Pot.
- Place the bundt pan on top of the trivet and close the lid.
- Cook at high pressure for 25 minutes.
- When the cooking is done, quick release the pressure and remove the lid.
- Carefully remove the cake from your Instant Pot and allow to cool for 10 minutes. Sprinkle powdered sugar over the cake. Serve and enjoy!

Nutrition information per serving:

- Calories: 291
- Fat: 11.6g
- Carbohydrates: 42g
- Dietary Fiber: 1g
- Protein: 4.7g

5. Enticing Pumpkin Chocolate Chip Bundt Cake
Time: 35 minutes
Servings: 8
Freestyle SmartPoints: 8
Ingredients:

- 1 ½ cups of all-purpose flour
- 1 teaspoon of pumpkin pie spice
- 1 teaspoon of ground cinnamon
- 1/4 teaspoon of salt
- ½ teaspoon of baking soda
- ½ teaspoon of baking powder
- ½ cup of butter softened
- 1 cup of sugar
- 2 large eggs, beaten
- 1 cup of pumpkin puree

- ¾ cups of mini-chocolate chips

Instructions:

- In a bowl, add the flour, pumpkin pie spice, cinnamon, salt, baking soda, and baking powder. Mix well.
- In another bowl, beat the butter and sugar until fluffy.
- Mix in the eggs one at a time.
- Add the pumpkin and mix until well combined.
- Add the flour mixture and mix until well combined.
- Fold in the chocolate chips.
- Grease a 6-cup bundt pan with nonstick cooking spray.
- Spoon the batter into the bundt pan. Tightly cover with aluminum foil.
- Add 1 ½ cup of water and a trivet inside your Instant Pot.
- Put the bundt pan on the trivet.
- Close and lock the lid. Cook at high pressure for 25 minutes.
- When the cooking is done, naturally release the pressure for 10 minutes and quick release any remaining pressure.
- Carefully remove the lid and carefully remove the bundt pan.
- Allow cooling for 10 minutes. Serve and enjoy!

Nutrition information per serving:

- Calories: 395
- Fat: 17.8g
- Carbohydrates: 55.4g
- Dietary Fiber: 2.3g
- Protein: 5.7g

6. Delightful Banana Chocolate-Chip Mini Muffins
Time: 10 minutes
Servings: 16
Freestyle SmartPoints: 4
Ingredients:

- 1 cup of vanilla yogurt
- ½ cup of fat-free skim milk
- 1/2 cup of quick oats

- ½ teaspoon of vanilla extract
- 1 large egg, beaten
- 1 large bananas, mashed
- 1 ¼ cup of all-purpose flour
- ¼ cup of brown sugar
- 2 teaspoons of baking powder
- ½ teaspoon of salt
- ½ teaspoon of baking soda
- ½ cup of mini-chocolate chips, divided

Instructions:

- In a bowl, add the milk, vanilla yogurt, vanilla extract, and eggs. Mix until well combined.
- Add the quick oats, bananas, flour, brown sugar, baking powder, salt, and baking soda. Stir until well combined.
- Fold in the chocolate chips.
- Add 1 cup of water and a trivet inside your Instant Pot.
- Using a cookie scoop, fill silicone muffins with the batter.
- Layer the muffin cups inside your Instant Pot. (Note: You may need to cook the muffins in batches if any leftover batter.)
- Cover the muffin cups with aluminum foil to prevent water from resting on top.
- Close and seal your Instant Pot.
- Cook at high pressure for 8 minutes.
- When the cooking is done, naturally release the pressure and remove the lid.
- Check if the muffins are done using a toothpick.
- Remove the muffins and allow to cool. Serve and enjoy!

Nutrition information per serving:

- Calories: 107
- Fat: 2.5g
- Carbohydrates: 17.7g
- Dietary Fiber: 0.9g
- Protein: 3.3g

Chapter Five

OCTAVIA PROGRAMS

alk to your healthcare provider about the programs and any medications or dietary supplements you are using, including, in particular, coumadin (warfarin), lithium, diuretics, or medications for diabetes, high blood pressure, or thyroid conditions, before starting a weight loss program. If you have a serious sickness (for e.g., cardiovascular disease including heart attack, cancer, diabetes, thyroid disease, liver or kidney disease, eating disorders such as anorexia or bulimia), or any other condition that requires medical care or that may be affected by weight loss, do not practice any Octavia program until you are allowed by your healthcare provider.

Choose the Best Program for You

The Teens Octavia plan is the only teens (13 to 17 years of age) suitable Octavia program. For seniors (65 years and older), teens, people with gout, nursing mothers, some people with diabetes, and those who exercise for more than 45 minutes per day, the Optimal Weight 5 & 1 Plan is not appropriate. If you fall into one of these categories above; please consult your healthcare provider and talk to your Octavia coach about other Octavia plans. Refer to our online program information, consult your healthcare provider, and talk to your Octavia coach for special medical or dietary needs, including food allergies. Do not take an Octavia product if you are allergic to any of the ingredients listed on the packaging of the product and on the website of Octavia for that product.

Each day, we recommend you to drink 64 ounces of water. Prior to changing the quantity of water you drink, consult with your healthcare provider as it can affect certain health conditions and medications.

NOTE: In some individuals, rapid weight loss may cause gallstones or gallbladder disease, or temporary thinning of hair. Some people may experience dizziness, headache, lightheadedness, fatigue, or gastrointestinal disturbances (such as abdominal pain, bloating, gas, constipation, diarrhea, or nausea) while adjusting to the consumption of a lower-calorie level and dietary changes. For further guidance on any other health care concerns, consult your healthcare provider. If you experience muscle cramps, tingling, numbness, confusion, or rapid/irregular heartbeat, seek immediate medical attention as these may be a sign of a more serious health condition.

In order to avoid doubt, the programs and products of Octavia shall not be labeled, advertised, or promoted for any specific medicinal purpose, i.e., for the treatment or prevention, implied or otherwise, of any disease or disorder, including the conditions associated with it.

Octavia programs, products, and any of their materials and information shall not constitute medical advice or a substitute for medical treatment in any way. As people may have different responses to dietary products or dietary changes, so talk to your healthcare provider about any medical concerns.

Why the 4 & 2 & 1 Plan for Optimal Weight?

If you prefer a flexible meal plan to help you to reach a healthy weight, The Optimal Weight 4 & 2 & 1 Plan is perfect for you. It can meet the needs of a broad variety of people. It is appropriate for you if you are:

Type 1 diabetes and are closely monitored by their provider of health care.

- Have Diabetes Type 2
- 65 years of age or older and are not regularly active
- Exercise in excess of 45 minutes a day
- Have to lose fewer than 15 pounds
- All food groups, including fruit, dairy, and starches, want to be integrated

It is as straightforward as this:

- Eat four carbs + 2 lean and green meals + 1 healthy snack *
- Eat six times a day, once every 2 to 3 hours,

One serving of starch, dairy fruit, or an Octavia Snack is a healthy snack. Refer to the Optimal Weight 4 & 2 & 1 Plan Guide for the full list.

The Optimal Weight 4 & 2 & 1 Plan, like all Octavia weight loss plans, emphasizes healthy habits such as portion control, exercise, drinking plenty of fluids, and eating small frequent meals.

On the Optimal Weight 4 & 2 & 1 Plan, what is the average weight loss?

The Optimal Weight 4 & 2 & 1 Plan encourages a steady, gradual loss of weight. Based on a numerous variables, such as starting weight, age, gender, adherence to the plan, and physical activity levels, to name a few, the amount of weight loss per week will vary from a person to person.

Octavia for Diabetes

Octavia provides meal plans that are suitable for the individuals with diabetes disease. For people with diabetes, meal planning is geared towards limiting calories while maintaining consistent, healthy levels of blood sugar.

The Octavia program is a great fit because, after every two to three hours, it incorporates tiny meals, so carbohydrates and protein are spaced throughout the day. And all of our fuels are controlled by carbohydrates and are generally lower in fat, making it a healthy option for people with diabetes disease.

All of our options for individuals with diabetes are outlined in the Octavia Diabetes Guide. Prior to start any weight loss program, we recommend that you should consult your healthcare provider. Talk to your healthcare provider about any medications, particularly Coumadin (warfarin), lithium, diabetes medications, or high blood pressure medications, when following a weight loss program.

It is particularly crucial for people with diabetes that your blood sugar levels should be carefully monitored throughout the weight loss process, as your medications may need to be adjusted, sometimes even before you start.

Octavia for Seniors

Achieving a healthy weight and learning healthy habits is a great way to boost your health and vitality for older adults. Three different meal plan options are included in our Octavia for Seniors plan, designed for adults 65 years and older.

In some cases, surgery alone may not be enough over the long term to maintain a healthy weight, and you may benefit from a calorie-controlled dietary meal plan. Octavia can help you accomplish and maintain your weight loss goals, regardless of the procedure you have undergone.

Octavia for Gout

Octavia offers a gout-specific plan that will help you reach a healthy weight. In order to provide about 1,200 calories per day, the Octavia for Gout Plan incorporates a balance of low purine foods, moderate protein, and two Octavia fuelings.

You will eat six times a day under this plan, after every two to three hours.

I have Polycystic Ovarian Syndrome (PCOS), and can I go on the Octavia program?

A hormonal disorder is common among women of reproductive age is a polycystic ovarian syndrome (PCOS). Usually, PCOS would not stop someone from following the Octavia program. In fact, for those with PCOS, the Octavia program may be particularly effective as it includes several PCOS treatment recommendations, such as achieving a healthy weight, incorporating regular exercise, taking an omega-three dietary supplement, and following a meal plan that is controlled by carbohydrates.

The Octavia program is created to help you to achieve your optimal weight while improving your health, trust, and vitality so that you can create space for a larger and more fulfilling life. Our most famous weight loss program is the Optimal Weight 5 & 1 Plan, but we also offer other programs to accommodate individual needs and preferences. To know more about our meal plan options, talk to your Octavia coach and then contact your healthcare provider before (and throughout) you start your journey with Octavia to discuss your health-related goals as they are related to the Octavia program.

In the First Few Days, What to Expect?

You may feel hungry, tired, or irritable as your body adjusts to a new way of eating as you begin with your journey to Optimal Wellbeing. This is temporary, but during this time, make sure you keep a close eye on your hunger. Have an extra fueling or a few extra ounces of lean protein (e.g., one hardboiled egg, 1-1.5 ounce reduced-fat cheese stick, etc.) if you're excessively hungry or tired in the first few days. It's better to have an additional Fueling than to go completely off from your program. These symptoms will disappear within a few days, leaving you to feel energized and confident. Remember, as you begin your journey, the support of your Octavia Coach will be so important, so do not hesitate to reach them if you have any questions or need additional support.

To make the modification and adjustment period easier, here are a few extra tips:

- Drink water and stay hydrated.
- Choose a start date if you do not expect any events focused on social food.
- Stay busy.
- Remind yourself that you are on a journey and take it one day at a time to enhance your health.
- Avoid temptations, and remain focused on your goals for health.

Each day, we recommend drinking 64 ounces of water. Before changing the amount of water, you drink, talk to your healthcare provider, as it can affect certain health conditions and medications.

What is Fat Burning?

The amount of protein you eat on the Optimal Weight 5 & 1 Plan is comparable to that found in a typical American meal plan. The quantity of carbohydrates, however, is lower compared to what typically can be consumed. As an individual, you can expect to take in less than 100 grams of total carbohydrates per day (usually in the range of 80-100 grams total) on the Optimal Weight 5 & 1 Plan.

In combination with the reduced-calorie level of the Optimal Weight 5 & 1 Plan, this lower level of carbohydrates allows your body to enter a fat-burning state. This is a gentle but efficient state of fat-burning which allows the body to achieve faster weight loss while helping to maintain muscle mass. The fat-burning state also helps to reduce appetite and hunger naturally while still allowing you to feel adequate energy levels. If you are in the fat-burning state, the best way to determine is to recognize physical indications such as feeling less hungry and more energized and losing weight at a steady rate.

How to Deal with Cravings?

Unhealthy food cravings are common and normal. They should be anticipated and it's not a sign of failure. Often times, cravings within ourselves or our environment are caused by signals. Physical problems such as tiredness, headaches, and hunger can spark cravings, negative emotional states such as stress, boredom, worry, and frustration, social or positive situations such as being at a holiday party or a restaurant.

Instead of trying to put pressure on it try to get it out of your head when we experience a craving, invite it in and try to understand it. Ask yourself, "Why now? How do I feel? Am I hungry? Am I Tired? Am I stressed? Once you understand the concerns behind your cravings, by avoiding or eliminating the signs that trigger them, you can try and avoid them."

To help you manage cravings, here are a few additional strategies:

Breathe Deep

Stopping and taking a few deep breath, cleansing breaths is one of the easiest and most powerful ways to handle as an unhealthy eating urge. Close your eyes and concentrate on calmly filling and emptying your lungs as your mind calms down, and your consciousness restarts. Open your eyes, and continue to enjoy yourself.

Distract Yourself

Switch gears if you think about food. Find an activity to distract your-self, such as calling a friend, taking a hot shower, or taking a walk.

The "Urge Surf"

It builds, crests crash gently on the shore, and sheds away into the sand. As interesting as the urge is, it's temporary: in a few minutes, you'll find that the feeling passes if you don't give in. A food craving is simply an ocean wave.

Walk It Out

Avoidance and physical activity give a practical one-two punch to food cravings. Remove yourself from temptation and take a walk, and then you will feel refreshed and re-energized again.

Talk It Out

Talking about the urge is to eat with someone who understands and can provide relief as you recognize that from time to time, it's not a sign of weakness or failure to have these feelings. Plus, as you stick to healthy choices, that person can give you valuable support.

Create A Healthy Setting

Remove all the temptations. Clean out any trigger foods from the refrigerator and cupboards, and instead store them with a healthy choices.

Counter-think

"When we worry that refusing food or drinks will hurt or offend some-one, or it will call attention to ourselves in a negative way, our inner dialogue can get us into trouble. Similarly, we may tell ourselves that if we have a bite of cake, it's all over, and we have failed to get healthy again in our attempt to get healthy. This negative self-talk can be counterbalanced by more constructive thoughts, such as," It's going to be more constructive.

Chapter Six

RELATIONSHIP WITH FOOD

*D*o you have a relationship with food that is healthy? It may sound like a question that is odd or superfluous. You don't have to worry about the emotions of your breakfast, whether you love your lunch or whether your dinner is about to break up with you.

But many people are struggling with an unhealthy relationship with food and dieting, says Erin Clifford, a Chicago-based wellness coach. For some people, by secretly consuming such diet-busting foods as chocolate chip cookies, muffins, ice cream, fried chicken, and hamburgers, that includes cheating on a diet. Some people eat emotionally, which is detrimental to maintaining a healthy lifestyle and losing unwanted pounds, to isolate themselves from their emotions. Because they are sad, stressed, bored, or lonely, people sometimes they eat. Typically, people who eat emotionally reach for unhealthy "comfort food," such as French fries or ice cream, which can lead to obesity, diabetes, and heart diseases.

Then there are people who are addicted to food, often to unhealthy things like chocolate, pizza, and chips for snacks. "Clifford says," Some people [are compulsive] about food, the same way some people are about alcohol or gambling. "Parallels exist."

But there is a food compulsion that differs from other conditions. For alcoholism and gambling, there are rehab centers and 12-step programs, but everyone needs to eat. Experts offer these tips and strategies to achieve and maintain healthy eating habits and prevent food from becoming an opponent or too-close friend:

1. Don't label good or bad for specific foods. There are no angelic health powers in a cup of broccoli, and a slice of pizza is not demonic. Some foods are much more essential than others for your well-being, but no food is either evil or benevolent, says Anne Lewis, an Indianapolis clinical psychologist at Indiana University Health.

Lewis says that ascribing moral qualities to foods gives them unwarranted power. That doesn't make you a bad person if you deviate from your diet and eat junk food, and you don't need to beat yourself up over it, which could lead to a sense of defeat and overeating. By understanding that some foods are more crucial for your health than others, maintain a healthy perspective on food, but no single type of food or portion will ensure or ruin your well-being.

2. Minimize your incentives to make bad decisions. It's OK to have a small piece of a cake on special events, such as your birthday or when you're out having dinner with friends, Lewis says, if you're on a low-sugar diet.

Limit the consumption of your cake to unusual events. Lewis says that keeping certain foods nearby can promote a habit of eating them, not keeping the cake in the home. Give it away or throw it out if you have a birthday celebration at your home, and you have leftover cake.

3. Don't get overly restrictive. Instead of completely cutting out certain foods, allow yourself to have a modest portion of your favorite treat one day a week. Instead of trying to banish donuts from your diet forever, for instance, allow yourself one in every seven days, says Clifford.

It might be unrealistic to try not to eat a specific food for the rest of your life. Instead of feeling like a failure, if you have that food, which could result in more binge eating, incorporate that food in moderation into your eating routine.

4. Keep your food diary. Write down not just about what you're eating, also write about what you feel at that time. Clifford advises that documenting your eating habits and emotions will assist you in detecting patterns.

You might see that when you feel sad, anxious, or depressed, you backslide from your good eating habits by consuming chips, cookies, or other junk foods. Try doing a little deep breath or going for a short walk instead of reaching for the unhealthy snack. "If you try that instead, your craving will pass a lot of times," Clifford says.

5. Just try cooking. Take the time to cook instead of heating up your meal in a microwave or picking up your food on the way home from a deli or fast-food joint. Make a list of delicious and healthy ingredients from the store that you need and enjoy choosing them.

You don't have to become a master chef. "Cooking can be a very simple," says Clifford. You can buy a steamer and toss it with your vegetables. Good indoor grills are available. If you go to the store to pick and prepare your ingredients, it makes you to appreciate your food more and it makes you mindful of it.'

6. At the grocery store, set yourself up for success. Dr. Michael Russo, a general surgeon who is specialized in bariatric surgery at the Memorial Care Center for Obesity at Orange Coast Memorial Medical Center in Fountain Valley, California, says that the battle to maintain a balanced and healthy relationship with food starts at the supermarket, where what you purchase will greatly determine whether you will maintain good and healthy eating habits.

In order to avoid aisles that are loaded with full of unhealthy items, your shopping trips can be strategized. "With cookies, crackers, snack chips, and other processed or refined foods high in carbohydrates, the last thing you want to do is load up your cart," Russo says. We are facing an obesity epidemic for the single most important reason. "Try shopping at the perimeter of the supermarket, where fresh produce, lean meats, dairy products, and baked items are sold, and avoid inside aisles, where snack items and sugar desserts are usually sold, Russo says." They are single most important reason why we are facing an obesity epidemic. Pick whole-grain bread and avoid cakes, muffins, and cookies when you are in the bakery section.

What is Orthorexia Nervosa?

Orthorexia is an eating disorder that is categorized by a healthy food obsession that is unsafe. An obsession with healthy, good dieting and consuming only "pure foods" or "clean eating" becomes deeply rooted in the way of thinking of the individual to the point that it interferes with their daily life.

Although orthorexia is not included in the Fifth Edition of the Diagnostic and Statistical Manual of Mental Disorders (DSM-5), many mental health professionals and eating disorder experts still recognize it and can have a harmful effect on their body, mind, and spirit.

Symptoms & Signs of Warnings

- Obsessions about ingredient checking.
- Fear of foods that are processed.
- Opting out for celebrations and social gatherings in fear of unhealthy foods that you may be forced to eat; demonstrates an "unusual interest" in what others eat.
- Inflexibility.
- Gluten-free.
- Inability to consume any food not designated "pure."
- Obsessively following bloggers or social media figures with a "healthy lifestyle."
- Checking nutrition labels or calorie counting compulsively.
- Perfectionism
- Veganism, Pescatarian or Vegetarian
- Dietary and nutritional supplement obsessions

Complications & Risks

Orthorexia can lead to a serious health problems, such as malnutrition, which can damage the kidneys and other vital organs, leading to a protein deficiency disorders. In addition, orthorexia is related to morbidity and mortality that can be increased by the presence of co-occurring disorders such as depression, anxiety, obsessive-compulsive disorder, and substance abuse disorders.

Causes of Anorexia Disease

- Personal conflicts unresolved.
- Previous history of trauma.
- Gastrointestinal issues, such as constipation, nausea, or bloating.
- Perfectionist character.
- Long Dieting History.
- Abuse of substances.
- Kidney troubles.
- Abnormalities of electrolytes such as low potassium, sodium, and chloride in the blood.
- Self-esteem low.
- Diminished testosterone in males.
- Unhealthy friendships.
- Obsession about exercise.

Treatment for Nervous Orthorexia

The approaches to psychotherapy offered in the treatment of eating disorder can allow an individual to recognize the underlying feelings and triggers associated with their orthorexia Nervosa and find strategies to develop a healthy mechanisms of coping and ways of living in reality without striving for perfection.

Orthorexia Nervosa leads to anorexia nervosa, which all of the mental health disorders, has the highest mortality rate. There are differences in treatment for orthorexia Nervosa alone or in combination with anorexia nervosa, as individuals with anorexia nervosa are focused on restoring weight during therapy.

Why Alcoholics Stay Lean After Ingestion of Calories

Nutritionists, who had long believed that every calorie that enter to the stomach could eventually turn into a fat, were baffled by that observation. Alcohol researchers wondered how the metabolic system, which millions of Americans knew was highly efficient in storing extra calories as fat, could waste so many alcohol calories.

Now Charles S. Lieber, a New York doctor since 1957 has been plumbing the depths of the many mysteries of alcohol, has come up with a biochemical mechanism that he says largely accounts for the remarkable waste of heavy drinkers' alcohol calories.

Lieber published his findings under the title 'Perspectives: Do Alcohol Calories Count?' in the Journal of the American Society for Clinical Nutrition.

The answer, he said, is yes and no: yes, for a moderate social drinker who has a pre-dinner cocktail or a glass of wine or a beer on a occasion. Alcohol calories can indeed add up for these individuals.

But certain metabolic processes can be primed by chronic heavy drinking and, in effect, train the body to waste the seven calories a gram that alcohol normally provides.

For instance, in alcoholics who were given 2,000 calories of alcohol daily on top of the 2,500 calories from the foods they consumed to maintain their weight, weight gain was negligible. But a steady weight gain resulted when the same amount of extra calories that was supplied as a chocolate.

Consequently, the energy waste associated with heavy alcohol intake cannot be attributed to a decrease in the intake of other foods. More probably, it results from interference with the ability of the body to obtain energy from other foods.

Experiments in laboratory animals and in heavy drinkers found that alcohol calories did indeed count for animals and people who consumed a very low-fat diet, according to Lieber's report.

For their metabolic inefficiency, Lieber cautioned that heavy drinkers pay a stiff price. This process allows their bodies to dissipate the calories of alcohol as useless heat and also converts a host of a substances that is transmitted by the environment and the food into chemicals that can seriously harm vital organs.

What Happens If You're Drinking Alcohol and Don't Eat?

The tendency for young women to skip meals was also confirmed by Dr. David Herber, director of the UCLA Center for Human Nutrition. Women do so, Herber also told the Los Angeles Times, in order to attend cocktail parties where they will probably consume high-calorie drinks.

"Drunkorexia" is not restricted, either, to the United States. A UK study has reported that 40 percent of young adults aged 25-34 have skipped their meals to save alcohol calories, according to Global News. Similarly, 34 percent of adults aged 18-24 have limited food for the same purpose, according to an Italian study.

Health professionals agree that this behavior is not healthy and has many risks.

Dr. Caroline Cederquist in Women's Health Magazine said, first of all, skipping meals and limiting calories have an opposite effect on weight than people think.

Cederquist is a specialist in weight management and the co-founder of bistroMD. According to her, skipping even a meal can slow your metabolism and can cause any food you eat with alcohol to get stored as a fat.

Moreover, these weight-conscious drinkers are likely later on to binge on alcohol and even food. That's due to the reduction in the blood sugar caused by limiting or skipping food, reports the Los Angeles Times.

The question goes deeper than weight, however. Susan MacFarlane, R.D., told Global News that alcohol consumed without food could lead to getting drunk faster. MacFarlane also noted that switching to alcohol from nutritious foods can lead to nutrient deficiencies.

Many young men and women may feel the need to continue this practice in spite of these risks. What many don't know is the increased danger they're putting themselves into.

The paper states in Barry's review that young adults account for

1,700 deaths associated with alcohol each year. Furthermore, hundreds of thousands suffer injuries related to alcohol, physical, and sexual assault.

Young adults only increase the odds of these situations happening to them by drinking on an empty stomach. You might even consider that they drink irresponsibly.

Imagine if it were as easy to eat as, say, refueling a car. Only when an indicator nudged toward E would you fill up, you might not be able to overdo it, or your tank would overflow, and you would never, ever dream of using it as a treat.

Instead, eating is anything but straightforward for many of us. What starts out as a biological necessity quickly gets entangled with different emotions, ideas, memories, and rituals. Food takes on all sorts of meanings, such as solace, punishment, appeasement, celebration, duty, and we may end up overeating, undereating, or eating unwisely, depending on the day and our mood.

I think it's time for us to think about our relationship with food, says Eve Lahijani, a Los Angeles-based nutrition health educator and dietician at UCLA. She offers three common steps to help get there.

1. Reconnect with your hunger.

So many things drive us to eat it's noon, and that means lunchtime, it's midnight, and that means snack time, we're happy, we're anxious, we'd rather not bring home leftovers, we're too polite to say no, we're bored, and oh, wow, has someone brought in donuts?!?

Similarly, we suppress our appetite for a myriad of reasons we're too busy, we're sad, we're mad, nobody else is eating, it's too early, it's too late, we're too excited.

Now try doing this: Eat only when you're hungry; stop when you're full. "It may seem obvious to you," Lahijani concedes. Think about your last week, though: How many times did you eat when you weren't starving?

She suggests that on a scale of 0-10, we think of our hunger and our fullness, with 0-1 being famished and 9-10 being painfully stuffed (as in stuffed holiday dinner). She says, "When you first get hungry, you want to start eating, and that correlates to three or four on the scale and [to stop] ... when you first get full, six or seven on the scale."

The reason you dare not to wait until you're starving is that when people tend to make nutritionally unsound choices (or 0-2 on the scale). You probably didn't fill up your basket with produce if you ever went to the supermarket when you were ravenous; you gravitated towards the high-calorie, super-filling items.

"Lahijani says," When you first get hungry, it's also wise to eat because you're more likely to enjoy your food [and] you're more likely to eat attentively. If you let yourself get very hungry, there are chances that you're eating really quickly and not really paying attention. Actually, letting yourself get too hungry in the first place is one of the biggest predictors of overeating.

2. Feed your body what it yearns for.

Her eating took one of two forms when Lahijani was a stressed-out college and graduate student: either she was dieting or bingeing. As she says: "The dietitian told me what to eat whenever I was on a diet,"; while on a binge, she would eat whatever was convenient or go all out on foods prohibited by her then. The development of a distinct food relationship meant stepping out of those patterns. She says, "Instead of listening to the views of others regarding what I should eat, I became silent and tuned into my own body." "I was feeding my body what it craved for."

Lahijani didn't crave for junk food, and it turns out. She says, "For the first time, I was actually tasting things because my mind was not filled with judgment and guilt." In fact, I discovered that my body craved nurturing, nourishing foods such as vegetables and fruits. Actually, I liked my sister's salad of kale and quinoa.

3. Do not treat food as a reward or punishment.

No wonder we're doing this. After all, as a children, we quickly learn that rejoicing and parties come with a cake, while transgressions result in no cake. But one of the great things about being an adult is that we can create associations of our own. Let's continue to mark our birthdays with a cake, by all means, or with fresh fruit and a stockpot of homemade veggie chili if you prefer that. Or, in many ways you can do that have nothing to do with eating to celebrate. From now you can set your own rules.

Habits of People with Food

Whether our particular problem is binge eating, emotional eating, disordered eating, or we just can't seem to get an idea on the whole nutrition thing, we can all stand to understand a few things from the people for whom the healthy eating just comes simple and easily. Here are some things they can do differently.

1. People with a good and healthy relationship to food eat mindfully.

Our body has some significant built-in cues to tell us when to eat and when to stop eating. But we're not always listening and concentrating to body. The practice of engaging all of our mind and senses to guide our eating decisions is called mindful eating, explains Megrette Fletcher, M.Ed., RD, CDE, current president of the Center for Mindful Eating. Mindful eating can aid us to "acknowledge our response to food without getting into judgment," she says.

2. They swear by all — yes, all — in moderation.

"No food is forbidden," says the clinical psychologist and the author of Emotional Eating, Edward Abramson, Ph.D. "Intrinsically, foods are not 'good' or 'bad.'" He tells an anecdote of a customer who once told him that French fries were the devil's job and it wasn't a joke. He says, "French fries are just French fries."

Morality attached to food may come from the fact that when it comes to food, he says, some religions have prohibitions to it. Take how "some foods are described as sinfully delicious," he says, for instance.

"It is not good or bad food. It is our experience," Fletcher says. "And that's not judging; it's categorizing." It can help inform your future choices by recognizing the food and eating situations that you find pleasant, she says. In contrast to, "I have to eat this way or those foods," she says, "people with a healthy relationship to a food say to themselves, "'Eating is an opportunity for me to nourish and nurture my well-being.'

3. But they know that the timing must be correct.

If you decide, however, that you're in the mood for fries or a pizza or a chocolate, Abramson says, enjoy your selection at a time when you're not hungry for a full meal, so you don't over eat it. "He says," If you're starving and then you're faced with your favorite food, you're going to consume a lot more of it. "Let's say, if you've got it for dessert, you've already had your meal, your stomach is full, you can really appreciate the chocolate sensations."

4. When they're physically hungry, they eat.

"Typically, emotional eating is intended to soothe unpleasant emotional excitement," says Abramson. "Unfortunately, he says, stress and anxiety often lead us to crave higher-calorie, fattier foods, and" most of us do not need extra caloric intake.

He adds that when we use food to try to soothe an emotion, we ask ourselves what that emotion tries to teach us instead of replacing it with regret or guilt for eating whatever we grabbed.

5. And when they're comfortably full, they stop eating.

Hunger and satiety, Fletcher says, both start small and grow larger and louder. "For Some of us, she says, don't hear hunger or fullness until it screams in our ears." But being more tuned-in while eating can also assist us to "hear" better. "Mindfulness is saying, 'I'm going to listen to my hunger harder and hear it when it's not screaming at me, and I'm going to listen to my fullness harder so it's not screaming at me [either].'" After every bite, both hunger and fullness change, so listening in can help you find the level of fullness where you can find to stop eat, she says.

6. It's breakfast they eat.

There is more energy for a regular breakfast eaters, better memories, and a lower cholesterol level. Overall, they also feel healthier and are usually leaner than their colleagues who don't eat a morning meal. "The key to healthy eating is to start your day with a healthy, balanced breakfast with proteins, fats, and carbs that is not high in sugar."

7. They do not keep in the house problematic foods.

Once you know your particular emotional eating patterns, says Abramson, you can take tiny steps to redirect them. One approach he recommends is not to keep particularly tempting food in the house anymore, so you could leave home to get a desert after dinner. If you love ice cream, for instance, "instead of having it sit in the freezer calling your name," he says, go out for a ice cream a couple of times in a week.

8. With the whole bag, they don't sit down.

Hitting up to your ice cream shop also has the benefit of offering a single serving size for your treatment. You know when you're done if you have a cup or a cone, you are opposed to sit there with one spoonful after another "straight out of the carton, Abramson says." It can also help to buy single serving packages of your favorite chips or cookies, he says, as you can simply serve yourself in a cup or a bowl instead of sitting down with a whole family sized chip bag.

9. Between a snack and a treat, they know the difference.

A recipe for overeating is to let yourself to get too hungry especially with those foods that you are willing to keep in smaller portions. Snacking is a clever way to ensure that you're not ravenous at a dinner time. But the choice of snacks is crucial for both keeping you full and keeping your healthy eating plans on track, Abramson says. "A treat is purely for pleasure, while a snack is something you eat to stave off hunger between meals," he says. "A good snack could be nuts, fruits or cheese," he says, but chocolate? Hey. A treat.

10. They permit themselves to enjoy eating.

When we don't make time to value our relationships with food, these tips are not plausible. "We forget to take our time to eat so many times, and eating takes time," says Fletcher. Instead of planning to scarf down something in the three minutes you have meetings in between afternoon, she suggests looking ahead to your day and making sure that you have enough time to eat. "We're doing it for three minutes, and it may feed you, but does it feeds you?" she asks. And by making time to eat, she says, it's not about feeling guilty for missing something else. This is really about believing that we are " worth to sit down and eat food."

11. They're not "making up" for a meal.

"There's this idea to make up for it by either overdoing it in the gym or being very restrictive at the next meal," says Cohn, when we find ourselves feeling guilty about a food choice. Instead, as a more subtle "balancing out," she suggests thinking of this process. For example, if they decide to indulge in a brunch, people with a healthy relationships with food will have a lighter meal later in that day, but they will not restrict that later meal so much that they end up binging late because they have made themselves excessively hungry. "Over the course of a week, you can balance out slowly, but you cannot make up within the same day," says Cohn.

12. They do not eat to see the shift in scale.

Ideally, we would all eat that what would make us feel good, Cohn says. Instead of restructuring our eating plans to change the number on the scale, we would pick the foods that gives us the energy to fuel our daily activity, and we would avoid foods that, give us indigestion, regardless of how good they are in taste.

13. They don't have any fear of feeling hungry.

Fear of eating a lot and consequently gaining weight is one of the most restrictive patterns of thought that Cohn has seen among the customers. "They are not as afraid of their hunger as people who have a sense of what their body needs and eat mindfully and intuitively when they can," she says. "What's there to be afraid of? If you're going to starve, you're just going to eat something!"

14. Their food worries do not interfere with everyday life.

Even the good eaters might feel a little overwhelmed after a long list of rules and habits like mentioned above. The key to a healthy acceptance of all this advice is to remain balanced. It can also cause problems to be too rigid, restrictive, or strict about nutritious eating, including disordered thoughts or conduct that could be categorized as orthorexia, says Cohn.

The one thing to schedule is a gym date, scheduling a date three nights in a row when your best friend is visiting from out of a town, and you don't take any time to see her, she says, may raise red flags. "In order to maintain a certain lifestyle, if you miss out any normal social engagements or sleep, that's definitely crossing the line."

Chapter Seven

OCTAVIA DIET RECIPES

What is a Lean and Green Meal?

- Lean and Green meals are a part of the Octavia program, and eating one of them per day is recommended.
- You can cook lean and green recipes for breakfast, lunch, or dinner, or in between, and make it your meal. It is really about what is going to work best for your timetable.
- Recipes that are lean and green consist of:

1. Approximately 6 to 7 ounces of cooked lean protein, such as fish, turkey, chicken breast, soy, or egg whites.
2. Up to 3 servings of vegetables that are not starchy, such as lettuce, celery, spinach, zucchini, or cucumbers.
3. Two healthy fat portions, such as avocado, olives, and olive oil.

What are Zoodles?

Zoodles are super-thinly cut zucchini that are cooked as a low carb replacement for pasta noodles.

Use Zoodles to cut out the carbs that is found in pasta for your Lean and Green recipes.

Can I have my Lean and Green Meal split?

Yes! Yes! You can divide the meal into two servings and eat half of it at a time.

I even used a meal and made it between the other main meals of the day for my snacks.

That's the beauty of protein and vegetables; they keep you full and stop you from snacking on those pesky carbs that are going to ruin out your diet.

How Do You Make Zoodles?

- Wash out the ends of the zucchini and slice them.
- Put the zucchini in a spiralizer and rotate the handle.
- Put parchment paper for a easy cleanup on a large baking sheet.
- Sprinkle sea salt on the zoodles lightly and spread it on the large baking sheet in a thin layer.
- Bake in the oven at approximately 350 degrees F for at least 15 min.

Lean and Green Garlic Chicken Zoodles

One of our favorite slim and green recipes is this creamy garlic chicken! Without guilt, it's colorful and packed with many flavors!

Cook Time15 mins
Prep Time15 mins
Total Time30 mins
Ingredients

- 1 1/2 lbs. boneless skinless chicken breasts
- 1/4 C parmesan cheese
- 1/2 tsp Italian seasoning
- 1 C spinach, chopped
- 3-6 slices sun-dried tomatoes
- 1/2 C chicken broth
- 1 C low fat plain Greek yogurt
- 1 1/2 C zucchini cut into thin noodles
- 1/2 tsp garlic powder
- 1 T olive oil
- 1 T chopped garlic

Instructions
How to Cook the Chicken?

1. Heat the oil in a large, medium skillet.

2. Pat the chicken breast dry, using paper towels, sprinkle with salt and pepper for the taste and place it in hot oil.

3. Cook on each side for 3-5 minutes on medium-high heat or until it is brown on each side and until the center is no longer pink.

4. Take the chicken out and keep it on a plate.

5. In a large skillet, add yogurt, chicken broth, garlic powder, Italian seasoning, and parmesan cheese.

6. whisk over medium heat, till it starts thickening.

7. Add the sun-dried tomatoes and spinach.

8. Simmer until it begins to wilt with the spinach.

9. Return the chicken to your pan and serve it over the zucchini noodles.

10. Make three servings for the

Per serve:

1 Leaner Protein

One fat

Three Seasonings

How are the Zoodles Cooked?

1. Preheat the oven to 350 ° F.

2. Trim the zucchini into the shape of spiral noodles using a vegetable spiralizer.

3. On a large baking sheet, place the parchment paper. Spread the zoodles and make them arrange, and toss them with a sea salt. Make sure they spread, so that they don't stick together.

4. Bake al dente for 15 min. Bake them more for a few minutes if you want them to be softer.

5. Serve immediately.

Nutrition

Serving: 1g | Carbohydrates: 8g | Saturated Fat: 4g |Calories: 414kcal | Cholesterol: 155mg | Protein: 60g | Fat: 15g

Breakfast Recipes

Lean & Green Muffinless Egg Cups

Prep time: 10 mins

Cook time: 13 mins

Total time: 23 mins

Serves: 4

Ingredients

- ½ tsp pepper or to taste
- 12 pieces of Canadian bacon (you can sub out for ham, BUT Canadian bacon is full of flavor and its pretty light)
- ¼ c chopped green chilies
- Four eggs
- One bunch green onions chopped
- 1 cup ripped spinach
- ⅛ tsp salt or to taste
- Eight egg whites

Instructions

1. Besides Canadian bacon, mix everything together. With a ¼ c measuring cup, fill muffin tins lined with the Canadian bacon, spray muffin tin and place Canadian bacon on the bottom. Bake for 13 minutes at 350 F.

Nutrition Information

Serving size: 3 cups

Protein: 22

Fat: 6.5

Calories: 163

Carbohydrates: 3.45

Lean & Green Omelet

Prep Time 10 minutes

Cook Time 5 minutes

Servings 1

Ingredients

- Two links Fully Cooked Turkey Breakfast Sausage, cut into 1/2-inch pieces
- **Two** eggs or four egg whites
- dash salt
- 2 tablespoons milk
- 1/4 cup swiss cheese or shredded mozzarella
- dash pepper
- 1/4 cup fresh baby spinach

Directions

1. Whisk the milk, eggs, salt, and pepper together in a small bowl. Coat the cooking spray with an 8-inch nonstick skillet. Heat until it is hot, over medium heat.

2. Pour the mixture of eggs into the skillet. Push cooked edges towards the center as the eggs cook, allowing uncooked portions to flow underneath.

3. Sprinkle the cheese, spinach, and sausage on one half of the omelet when the eggs are set. Halve the folding omelet.

4. Cook for 1 minute again or until the cheese is melted. Put the omelet on the plate.

Proteins 22g

Carbohydrate 2.25g

Fats 5.5g

Calories 185cal

Poultry Recipes

Chicken Francaise

Prep time: 15 minutes

Cook time: 20 minutes

Total time: 35 minutes

Servings: 4

Ingredients

- Two tablespoons lemon zest
- One teaspoon pepper
- ½ cup flour
- ¼ cup olive oil
- Two tablespoons parmesan cheese
- Two large eggs
- Four chicken breasts pounded with a meat mallet until it gets thin
- One teaspoon salt
- ½ lemon, juiced
- ½ cup white wine
- Two tablespoons butter
- 1 cup chicken broth
- One tablespoon flour
- 454 grams of pasta
- Four tablespoons fresh parsley
- Two tablespoons minced red peppers
- 2-3 tablespoons minced white onion
- ½ cup canned artichoke hearts, drained

Instructions

1. Combine the coating components in a bowl.

2. First, dip the chicken in your flour mixture. Then dip the beaten egg into it. Then return to the mixture of flour for another coating. Give time to let them sit for a minimum of 15 minutes in the fridge.

3. Heat oil over medium-high heat in a large skillet. Cook the chicken on each side for 4-5 minutes, cook it until it reaches to 165 ° F. Remove from the skillet and place on a clean plate once its done.

4. If you use my add-ins, fry the onions and red peppers until they are tender and cook it in the 2 tbsp of butter at this time. Stir the flour along with the vegetables into the skillet.

5. If the added vegetables are not used, melt the butter in the skillet, and then add the flour.

6. Add the wine to the skillet slowly and begin to scrape the browned bits into the mix. (Make it deglaze). The lemon juice and the chicken broth are whisked in. Simmer for 4-5 minutes on a medium-high heat, for further reducing the sauce.

7. Return the chicken breasts to the sauce and heat them again. If you want the artichoke and the capers, add them at this point to heat up.

8. Serve with fresh parsley over your choice of pasta and top.

Protein: 30g

Fat: 25 g

Saturated fat: 7g

Calories: 447cal

Carbohydrates: 16g

Cholesterol: 194mg

Fried Chicken Strips

Prep time: 30 minutes

Servings: 4

Ingredients

- Two large eggs
- ¾ cup flour
- One teaspoon paprika
- ½ cup panko crumbs
- Four medium chicken breasts
- Two teaspoons garlic powder

- 1 ½ tablespoons seasoning salt
- One teaspoon pepper

Instructions

1. Cut your chicken breasts lengthwise into strips. You don't need them to be more than 1/2 an inch thick, so they're not going to cook. You can take a meat mallet, if necessary, to the strips to flatten them. 4-6 strips will be made for each breast.

2. In a medium-sized bowl, whisk together the first six ingredients.

3. In a small bowl beat the eggs.

4. Get a big sheet for baking and line it with parchment paper.

5. First, dip your chicken strips and cover them completely in the flour crumb mixture.

6. For a second coat, dip it into the egg mixture, then into the flour crumb mixture again.

7. Place the baking sheet on it.

8. Repeat with all pieces of the chicken.

9. For half an hour, place the baking sheet in the refrigerator.

10. Preheat to 365 ° F a deep skillet of oil.

11. Place each tender chicken in the oil, leave space between them, and cook them in batches. Cook on each side for 2-3 minutes, turn them until each tender is browned on the outside and make them fully cooked to a minimum of 165 ° F in the middle.

12. On a plate lined with paper towels, remove and place.

13. Until they are finished, repeat cooking the tenders.

14. Serve with the sauce for dipping.

Protein: 55g

Carbohydrates: 25g

Calories: 416cal

Fat: 9g

Saturated fat: 2g

Snack and Appetizer

Banana Oatmeal Muffins

Prep Time: 35 mins

Servings: 4

Ingredients:

Muffin Batter:

- 1/2 teaspoon baking soda

- 1 1/2 cups all-purpose flour
- 3/4 cup sugar
- 1/2 teaspoon salt
- 1 cup quick oats
- Two teaspoons baking powder
- 1/2 cup vanilla low-fat yogurt
- 1 1/2 cups very ripe bananas
- 1/4 cup vegetable oil
- One large egg, slightly beaten
- 1/4 Teaspoon nutmeg

Topping:

- 1/4 cup chopped pecans
- 1/4 cup old fashioned oats
- 2 Tablespoons flour
- 1 Tablespoon butter softened
- 1/4 cup light brown sugar
- 1/4 Teaspoon cinnamon

Muffin Baking Tips for the Banana Oatmeal Muffins

As soon as your batter is mixed together, spoon the muffin batter into the pan. As soon as the batter is produced, the leavening will begin, and you want that to happen in the oven.

Have you ever made muffins and discovered before baking them that you have a few empty muffin tins without batter? To prevent the tin from warping during baking, place two to three tablespoons of water in the empty muffin tins before baking.

A black metal pan more quickly absorbs and distributes heat than the lighter-colored pans. In a black colored pan, your muffins will bake faster and run the risk of burning if the heat that is reduced by 25 degrees. Suppose you bake with dark-colored pans and start checking your muffins with a toothpick 10 minutes before the recipe bake time is on the safe side.

Recipe for Banana Oatmeal Muffins- Before You Start

We will preheat the oven to 375 degrees before we begin the recipe and line a 12-cup muffin tin with paper liners. If you're not using paper liners, shorten the muffin tin by greasing it. Just like every muffin recipe, we start the muffin recipe by placing in one bowl the wet ingredients and in another bowl the dry ingredients. In the medium bowl, mix the wet ingredients: low-fat vanilla yogurt, egg, vegetable oil, mashed bananas, sugar, and quick oatmeal. The ingredients are whisked together and set aside for 10 minutes. Recall that we have quick oats in the bowl, and they need a little time to soften up. Why should we set it aside for ten minutes?

Combining the Components

In the large bowl, mix the dried ingredients: flour, baking powder, baking soda, salt, and nutmeg, and whisk them to combine. Use your fingers to place the topping ingredients into a small bowl, work the ingredients together until they are crumbly, and then set them aside.

It's time for the wet and dry ingredients to be combined. Add the dried ingredients to the wet ingredients and stir until the ingredients are mixed. While mixing with a wooden spoon, this will require about 15 to 20 strokes. "Just combined" implies that the dry ingredients are no longer dry, period. A muffin batter is an entirely different kind of animal than a cake batter. Your goal with a cake batter is to beat it until it's smooth, mixing a muffin batter only until the batter's ingredients come together with tiny lumps in the batter. Why do we not combine the wet and dry ingredients together using an electric mixer? It's too easy to use an electric mixer to overmix a muffin batter.

Fill the 3/4 full muffin tins with batter. Sprinkle the topping over the muffin batter and bake for 20 -25 minutes or until it is set and browned on top in a 375-degree oven. If you can wait that long, remove the muffins from the oven to a cooling rack and cool them for 15 minutes!

Berry Honey Yogurt Parfait
Prep time: 10 mins
Servings: 2
Ingredients

- 1 cup granola divided
- Four tablespoons honey divided
- Three tablespoons Carnation Breakfast Essentials Powder in French Vanilla
- 2 cups vanilla Greek yogurt divided
- 1 cup of mixed berries such as raspberries, strawberries, and blueberries

Instructions

1. Combine the blended berries and the Carnation Breakfast Essentials Powder in the French Vanilla in a medium bowl. Just set aside.

2. On top of two glasses or small bowls spread 1/2 cup of yogurt on the bottom.

3. Put 1/4 cup of granola on top, followed by one tablespoon of honey and 1/4 cup of mixed berries. With the second layer in each glass, repeat it.

Fish and Seafood Recipes
Spicy Tuna and Avocado Fish Taco
Cook Time: 15 mins
Prep Time: 20mins
Total Time: 35 mins
Ingredients

- Juice of 1 lime, and add lime wedges for serving
- Pickled red onions
- Salt and black pepper to taste
- 1/2 Tbsp canola or olive oil
- One ripe avocado, pitted, peeled, and sliced
- Hot sauce
- 2 Tbsp olive oil mayonnaise
- 12 oz fresh ahi or other high-quality tuna
- Eight corn tortillas
- 4 cups shredded red or green cabbage
- 1/2 Tbsp canned chipotle pepper

Instructions

1. In the large mixing bowl, mix the cabbage, mayo, lime juice, and chipotle together.

2. With salt and pepper, season. Put that slaw aside. (At least 15 minutes before cooking; this is best done so that you can allow the flavors to marry.

3. Heat the oil over a medium-high heat in a large cast-iron skillet or stainless-steel sauté pan.

4. With a salt and plenty of black pepper, season the tuna.

5. Add the tuna and sear on each side for 2 minutes when the oil is hot until a nice crust has developed, but the tuna inside is still rare.

6. Heat the tortillas until it is lightly crisp on the outside while the pan is still hot.

7. Cut your tuna into thin planks.

8. Divide the tortillas and top each one with slices of avocado, slaw, and pickled onions.

9. Use lime wedges and hot sauce to serve.

Calories: 330

Fat: 13g

Saturated fat: 2g

Serves: 4

Grilled Swordfish with Caponata
Prep time: 20 mins
Cook time: 15 mins
Servings: 2
Ingredient

- Two medium eggplants, slice into 1⁄2" cubes
- 1 Tbsp sugar
- Two cloves garlic, minced
- Salt and black pepper to taste
- 2 Tbsp raisins (preferably golden raisins)
- 2 Tbsp capers
- Four small swordfish steaks, 6 oz each
- One medium onion, diced
- 2 Tbsp red wine vinegar
- One can (14 1⁄2 oz) diced tomatoes
- 1⁄4 cup chopped fresh basil
- 1 Tbsp of olive oil, and add more for coating the fish

Instructions

1. Heat olive oil over a medium heat in a medium saucepan.

2. Add the eggplant, onion, and garlic, and sauté until it is lightly browned and softened for about 5 minutes.

3. Add tomatoes, raisins, vinegar, capers, and sugar.

4. Cover and steam it till the vegetables are very soft, and the mixture is marmalade like for 15 minutes.

5. Stir in the basil and add the salt and black pepper to the seasoning. Just stay warm.

6. At a medium-high heat, preheat a grill or grill pan.

7. Coat your swordfish with olive oil and season it with a salt and black pepper on the both sides. Grill the steaks for 4 minutes until they have

developed nice grill marks (you can rotate the steaks 45 degrees in the middle to make diamond-shaped grill marks if you like).

8. Flip and continue to cook until the flesh flakes with gentle pressure from your finger, for about 4 minutes longer.

9. With a generous scoop of caponata above the top, serve each serving of swordfish.

calories: 360

fat: 11g

saturated fat: 2.5g

servings: 4

Easy Creamy Cajun Shrimp Pasta

Prep time: 30 mins

Servings: 2

Ingredients:

- 1/2 c. heavy whipping cream
- 8 oz linguine pasta
- 1/2 c. chopped red peppers
- 1/2 c. unsweetened almond milk
- One Tbsp Cajun seasoning is divided into 1/2 Tbsp servings. You can also use creole seasoning.
- 1 lb. raw shrimp, deveined and removed shells.
- 1/2 c. chopped green peppers
- 2 tsp olive oil Divided into one teaspoon per servings.
- 1/2 c. shredded Parmesan Reggiano Cheese
- 1/2 c. chopped yellow or white onions
- 4 oz andouille sausage Sliced into 1-inch pieces. You can use more if you like.
- 4 oz cream cheese Cut into chunks.1 c. fire-roasted diced tomatoes Drained from a can.
- 1 Tbsp butter

Directions:

1. As per package instructions, cook the pasta.

2. Along with 1/2 Tbsp of cajun or creole seasoning, place the shrimp in a bowl. To guarantee that the shrimp is fully coated, mix it.

3. On a medium-high heat, heat a skillet or pan. I use a skillet that is made up of cast iron. To the pan, add one teaspoon of olive oil.

4. Add the shrimp to the pan when its hot. Cook on each side for 2-3 minutes until it turns bright pink. Remove and set aside the shrimp.

5. Along with the chopped sausage, onions, green peppers, and red peppers, add an additional teaspoon of olive oil to the pan.

6. Saute the vegetables till they are soft and the onions are translucent and fragrant, for 3-4 minutes. Remove and set aside the vegetables from the pan.

7. Reduce the heat to medium in the pan. To the pan, add the butter and allow it to melt.

8. Add heavy cream, almond milk, cream cheese, 1/2 tablespoon of the remaining Cajun or Creole seasoning, and the Reggiano parmesan cheese.

9. Continue stirring the sauce until it has completely melted all of the cheese. It may take some time for the cream cheese to melt. Add the roasted tomatoes to the fire and stir them. Allow 2 minutes to cook the mixture.

10. Mix and stir in the shrimp, sausage, vegetables, and pasta in the pan. Allow the pasta to cook, until it is combined, for 4-5 minutes. Then just serve.

Calories: 384

Fat: 22g

Protein: 7g

Carbohydrate: 22g

Servings: 2

Lean Meat Recipes
Quick and Easy Mongolian Beef
Prep time: 30 mins
Servings 4
Ingredients:

- One yellow onion sliced
- 2-4 Tbsp canola oil
- 2 Tbsp cornstarch
- ¼ c. low sodium soy sauce
- 1 lb. flank steak thinly sliced against the grain
- Two green onions chopped, and make green and white parts separated
- 3 Tbsp brown sugar
- Four garlic cloves chopped
- 1- inch ginger chopped

- ¼ c. water
- 1 Tbsp hoisin sauce
- Salt to taste

Directions:
1. Cover the flank steak with cornstarch, making sure each piece is fully covered. Just set aside.

2. Heat the canola oil at a medium heat in a large skillet. Once the oil is hot, add the flank steak in a single layer to the frying pan, making sure that the pieces do not touch eachother. Cook it until each side is browned for 1-2 minutes per side. Cook until all the flank steak is cooked in batches. Just set aside.

3. Add the sliced yellow onion, green onion whites, garlic, and ginger to the skillet and fry for approximately 3 minutes until the onions are slightly softened but they are still crunchy. Add soy sauce, water, brown sugar, and hoisin sauce and stir. Along with the green portions of the onions, add the steak back to the pan.

Take it out from the heat and serve.

Calories 303g

Fat 13g

Saturated fat 3gprotein 26g

Carb 20g

Vegetable Recipes
Grilled Chicken and Vegetable Shish Kebab
Prep time 20 mins
Cook time 15 mins
Servings 4
Ingredients:

- One orange bell pepper
- 2 Tbsp Better Than Bouillon roasted chicken base
- One red bell pepper
- One green bell pepper
- 2 lb. boneless chicken breasts
- One whole zucchini
- 8 oz cubed pineapples
- 2 tsp oregano
- 2 tsp black pepper
- 2 tsp paprika

For the teriyaki pineapple sauce:

- 2 Tbsp fresh pineapple juice
- 1/2 c. low-sodium soy sauce
- 2 tsp cornstarch
- 2 tsp Sesame Oil
- 2 tsp minced garlic
- 1/4 tsp Himalayan salt
- 1 tsp black pepper
- 1/4 tsp garlic powder
- 2 Tbsp brown sugar

Directions:

1. Start by starting the grill with your fire and allow the temperature to reach 350 degrees.

2. Cut the chicken breast into little cubes and put it in a large bowl. Rub the ingredients into the chicken and season the chicken with oregano, black pepper, and paprika.

3. To the chicken, add Better Than Bouillon roasted chicken base. Then mix well together and set to the side.

4. Remove each of the bell peppers from the stem and seeds and cut them into large pieces. In slices, chop the zucchini.

5. In the desired order, place each ingredient individually on the skewers.

6. Place every skewer of chicken and veggie on the grill. Grill on each side for 4 minutes. Then take out from the heat.

7. For the sauce, on medium / high heat, add all the ingredients in a small cooking pan until it begins to bubble, then reduce the heat to simmer and cook for 8 minutes and remove it from the heat and allow it to cool.

8. Immediately serve.

Calories 408g

Fat 6g

Saturated 0.4g

Carb 34g

Protein 56.7g

Vegan Recipes

Vegan Chorizo Tostadas

Prep time 15 mins

Cook time 15 mins
Servings 4
Ingredients:

- 2 Tbsp of vegetable oil
- Four c. of shaved Brussels sprouts
- Mexican crema (I use cashew cream)
- 1 / 2 tsp salt
- 1 / 2 tsp of ground cumin
- One avocado sliced
- Pinch of ground cloves
- 2 Tbsp of chili powder ground dried chili powder
- 1 / 4 tsp freshly pepper
- 12 corn tostada shells
- 1 tsp of garlic powder
- 1 / 8 tsp ground cinnamon
- 1 / 2 tsp apple cider vinegar
- 1 c. refried beans

Directions:

- Over a medium heat in a skillet.
- Be careful that they are not burned. Remove from the heat, when they are ready, and add the vinegar. Blend and set aside.
- To put the tostadas together, add two tablespoons of refried black beans and spread them well throughout the tostada.
- Then add the potent vegan chorizo, aka, the Brussel sprouts with Mexican spices, three or four tablespoons.
- Finish with slices of avocado for each tostada and drizzle with cashew or tofu cream.

Calories 268
Fat 11g
Saturated fat 4g
Protein 7g
Carb 37g
Soup Recipe
Spicy Korean Beef Noodle Soup
Prep time 20 mins

Cook time 15 mins
Servings 4
Ingredients:

- 2 Tbsp toasted sesame oil
- 1.7 oz mung bean noodles (sometimes called cellophane or glass noodles)
- 1 ½ - 2 Tbsp Korean red pepper flakes
- 4 c. Rich Beef Broth
- 1 c. water
- Fish sauce or soy sauce for serving
- 2 c. bok choy chopped
- Extra Korean red pepper flakes for serving
- Four fresh shitake mushrooms sliced
- Two scallions cut into 2" lengths
- 1 c. cooked short rib meat shredded (from rich beef broth recipe)

Directions:
1. For 20-30 minutes, soak mung bean noodles in hot water; drain.

2. In a small pan, heat sesame oil, red pepper flakes, and garlic until it is fragrant and light brown with garlic; mix with shredded meat; set aside.

3. Heat the beef broth in a large saucepan with the water. Add bok choy, mushrooms, and drained soaked mung bean noodles; cook until noodles are soft and bok choy is cooked about 3-4 minutes. To soup and heat through, add marinated meat and scallions. Divide between bowls; for spicy food lovers, serve with extra Korean red pepper flakes. Serve with fish sauce or soy sauce on the side for a drizzle if the beef broth is unsalted.

Calories 314
fat 8g
saturated fat 5g
protein 22g
carb 18g

Crockpot Beef Vegetable Soup
Prep time 20 mins
Servings 4
Ingredients:

- 1 Tbsp extra virgin olive oil
- 3-4 c. low sodium beef broth divided
- One small yellow onion diced
- Two parsnips peeled and diced
- Two cloves garlic minced (about 2 tsp)
- ¼ tsp black pepper
- 2 tsp kosher salt divided
- Four large carrots peeled them and finely chopped
- 2 Yukon gold potatoes peeled and diced
- Two ribs celery diced
- Chopped fresh parsley that is optional for serving
- 1 lb. boneless chuck roast or beef stew meat cut into 1-inch cubes
- ½ tsp smoked paprika
- One can tomato sauce (8 ounces)
- ½ tsp granulated sugar
- 3 Tbsp tomato paste
- 1 Tbsp Worcestershire sauce
- 1 tsp dried oregano
- One 14.5-ounce can of diced tomatoes
- 1 c. peas fresh or frozen (no need to thaw)

Directions:

1. Heat the oil in a large skillet over a medium heat. Add one teaspoon of the salt and pepper to the beef and sprinkle over it. On all sides, brown the beef, disturbing it as little on each side as possible so that it creates nice coloring. Remove it to a 6-quart slow cooker once the beef is lightly browned (it won't be cooked all the way through).

2. Add the onion to the pan. Cook and stir for about 3 minutes, until the onion begins to soften. Add the garlic and let it cook for 30 seconds. Splash the beef broth in about 1/2 cup and scrape up any browned bits that have stuck to the bottom (it's flavor!). For 2 minutes, let the broth decrease and then transfer the entire mixture to the slow cooker.

3. Carrots, potatoes, parsnips, celery, diced tomatoes, tomato sauce, tomato paste, Worcestershire, oregano, paprika, sugar, 2 1/2 cups of beef broth, and the remaining one teaspoon of salt are added to the slow cooker.

4. Cover and steam until the beef and vegetables are tender, on low, for 8 hours. Stir in the peas until they're warmed up. Add the remaining 1 cup

of beef broth until you reach your desired consistency if the soup is thicker than you want. Serve hot, with fresh parsley sprinkled on top.

Calories 283

Fat 7g

Saturated fat 2g

Protein 24g

Carb 33g

Meat Recipe

Meat and Rye Panzanella

Prep time 15 mins

Cook time 15 mins

Servings 4

Ingredients:

- 2 tbsp. red wine vinegar
- 2 tsp. caraway seeds
- One clove garlic, pressed
- Three slices rye bread (1 inch thick)
- 4 tbsp. olive oil, divided
- One bulb fennel, quartered
- Kosher salt and pepper
- 1 lb. sirloin steak
- One medium red onion, sliced into rounds
- 1 tbsp. whole-grain mustard
- One large bunch of chopped kale leaves (about 10 cups)

Directions:

1. Toast the caraway seeds in a small, medium skillet for about 2 minutes. Whisk the vinegar together, two tablespoons of oil, mustard, garlic, caraway seeds, and 1/4 teaspoon of salt in a small bowl.

2. Heat a medium-high grill or a barbecue pan. Brush 1 tablespoon of oil with the fennel, onion, bread and season with the fennel and onion with a pinch of a salt. Covered the Grill, often turning, until vegetables are soft and well-cooked and bread is toasted, 5 to 8 minutes for vegetables and 1 to 2 minutes for bread. Transfer to cutting board; fennel and tear bread into chunks, core, and thinly slice.

3. Toss the kale, grilled vegetables, and bread in a large bowl with half the dressing and let it sit, tossing occasionally.

4. Rub the steak with the remaining one tablespoon of olive oil and

season with 1/2 teaspoon of salt and pepper each time. Grill to the desired doneness, medium-rare for 4 to 6 minutes per side. Transfer to the cutting board and leave to rest before slicing for 5 minutes. Fold in the salad and drizzle with the vinaigrette leftover.

Carb 28g

Calories 435

Fat 23g

Saturated fat 5g

Protein 29g

Sandwich Recipe

Peanut Butter and Banana Sandwich

Prep time 20 mins

Servings 2

Ingredients

- Sliced banana – 1 medium (109 calories)
- Blueberries – 3/4 cup (61 calories)
- Peanut butter – 1 tablespoon (96 calories)
- Whole wheat bread – two slices (138 calories)

Preparation

1. On two toasted bread slices, spread peanut butter.
2. Top with banana slices and blueberries on the slices.
3. Eat open-faced with them.

Weight Loss Benefits

- Whole wheat bread is rich in fiber that provides satiety and regulates weight gain. Whole grains increase the time of chewing, which reduces the rate of eating and reduces the intake of energy.
- Protein-rich peanut butter. -1 tablespoon of peanut butter has at least 4 g of protein in it. It also helps to decrease the danger of type 2 diabetes.
- Adding fruit to sandwiches can provide essential vitamins and minerals for your body. They are lower in calories and higher in fiber and help regulate the gain in weight.

Tuna Salad Toast

Ingredients

- Lettuce cold cut leaves – one leaf inner (1 calorie)
- Whole grain bread – two slices (138 calories)
- Tuna salad from a deli counter – ½ cup (192 calories)
- Mayonnaise (Light, cholesterol-free) – one tablespoon (49 calories)

Preparation
1. From the local deli, pick up a cup of tuna salad.
2. Spread it out on toasted slices of bread.
3. Add the mayonnaise and lettuce leaves and enjoy the sandwich.

Weight Loss Benefits

- Tuna has low-calorie content. -1 oz. (28 g) contains only 31 calories and 7 g of satiety-providing protein.
- Combining tuna with whole wheat bread makes it a healthy, healthy, and perfect breakfast combo. It is rich in satiety-providing protein, fiber, and complex carbohydrates.
- Lettuce has a very low amount of calories and is suitable for the loss of weight.

Dessert Recipes
Zucchini Chocolate Chips Cookies
Prep time 20 mins
Cook time 10 mins
Total time 30 mins
Ingredients

- 1/4 tsp. baking soda
- 1 1/2 c. all-purpose flour
- 1 tsp. vanilla extract
- 1/2 c. packed brown sugar
- 1/4 tsp. kosher salt
- 1 c. old-fashioned oats
- One large egg
- 5 tbsp. butter softened
- 1/4 tsp. ground cinnamon
- 1/2 c. granulated sugar
- 1/4 c. plain Greek yogurt
- 1 c. shredded zucchini

- 1 c. semi-sweet chocolate chips

Directions
For Oven

1. Preheat the oven to 350 degrees. Whisk the flour, salt, baking soda, and cinnamon together in a small bowl.

2. Whip the sugar and butter together in a large bowl until it gets light and fluffy. Combine the egg, yogurt, vanilla and mix until it combined evenly. Mix the flour mixture until it's just mixed. Use oats, chocolate chips, and zucchini to fold in. Place on baking sheets with a rounded teaspoon with 2 inches apart.

3. For 15 minutes, bake. Cool it on the baking sheet for at least 2 minutes and transfer it to the wire rack to cool it completely. Note: Cookies are going to spread a little bit but does not take on a lot of colors.

For Air Fryer

1. Whisk the flour, salt, baking soda, and cinnamon together in a small bowl.

2. Whip the sugar and butter together in a large bowl until it gets light and fluffy. Combine the egg, yogurt, and vanilla and mix it until combined evenly. Mix the flour mixture until it's just mixed. Use oats, chocolate chips, and zucchini to fold in.

3. Air fryer liner basket with parchment paper. Use the small cookie scoop to scoop dough to work in batches and place at least 1 inch apart on parchment paper.

4. Cook for 10 minutes at 350 °?! Remove cookies and keep it to cool and repeat with remaining dough on a wire rack. Note: Cookies are not going to spread much but are going to get golden brown.

Chapter Eight

KIDNEY-FRIENDLY KITCHEN STAPLES

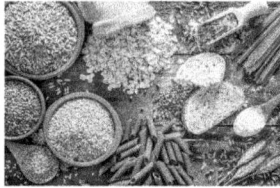

Kidney-Friendly Kitchen Staples

1. **BBQ Rub for Chicken**
   Preparation Time: 5 minutes
Cooking Time: 0 minutes
Servings: 3 tablespoons, ¾ tablespoons per serving
Ingredients:

- 1 teaspoon onion powder
- 1 teaspoon garlic powder
- ⅛ teaspoon ground red pepper
- 1 teaspoon red chili powder
- 1 tablespoon brown sugar
- ¼ teaspoon dry mustard powder
- ⅛ teaspoon allspice
- 1 teaspoon smoked paprika
- 1 teaspoon cumin

Directions:

1. Take a medium bowl, place all the ingredients in it, and stir well until combined.

2. Transfer the rub to an air-tight glass container and store until ready to use.

3. Sprinkle the rub all over the chicken piece and cook as instructed in the recipe.

Nutrition:
Calories: 20, Carbs: 4 g, Sodium: 9 mg, Potassium: 34 mg, Phosphorus: 7 mg

2. Cajun Seasoning
Preparation Time: 5 minutes
Cooking Time: 0 minutes
Servings: 5 tablespoons, 2 ½ tablespoons per serving
Ingredients:

- 4 teaspoons onion powder
- 4 teaspoons garlic powder
- 4 teaspoons paprika
- 2 teaspoons cayenne pepper

Directions:

1. Take a medium bowl, place all the ingredients in it, and stir well until combined.

2. Transfer the rub to an air-tight glass container and store until ready to use.

Nutrition:
Calories: 25, Carbs: 5 g, Protein: 1 g, Fiber: 1 g, Sodium: 15 mg, Potassium: 36 mg, Phosphorus: 5 mg

3. Chinese Five-Spice Blend
Preparation Time: 5 minutes
Cooking Time: 0 minutes
Servings: ¼ cup, 1 teaspoon each serving
Ingredients:

- ½ teaspoon ground allspice mix
- 6 teaspoons ginger powder
- 1 teaspoon ground cloves
- 1 tablespoon ground cinnamon

- ½ teaspoon anise seed

Directions:

1. Take a medium bowl, place all the ingredients in it, and stir well until combined.
2. Transfer the rub to an air-tight glass container and store until ready to use.

Nutrition:
Calories: 20, Carbs: 4 g, Fiber: 1 g, Sodium: 14 mg, Potassium: 49 mg, Phosphorus: 4 mg

4. Taco Seasoning
Preparation Time: 5 minutes
Cooking Time: 0 minutes
Servings: ½ cup, 1 tablespoon per serving
Ingredients:

- 1 tablespoon onion powder
- 1 teaspoon garlic powder
- ¼ cup red chili powder
- 1 teaspoon crushed red pepper
- 1 tablespoon ground cumin
- 1 teaspoon dried oregano
- ½ teaspoon cinnamon

Directions:

1. Take a medium bowl, place all the ingredients in it, and stir well until combined.
2. Transfer the rub to an air-tight glass container and store until ready to use.

Nutrition:
Calories: 14, Carbs: 3 g, Protein: 1 g, Fiber: 1 g, Sodium: 3 mg, Potassium: 34 mg, Phosphorus: 9 mg

5. Mexican Blend
Preparation Time: 5 minutes
Cooking Time: 0 minutes

Servings: ½ cup, 2 tablespoons per serving
Ingredients:

- 1 tablespoon onion powder
- 1 teaspoon garlic powder
- 1 teaspoon crushed red pepper
- ¼ cup red chili powder
- 1 tablespoon ground cumin
- 1 teaspoon dried oregano
- ½ teaspoon cinnamon

Directions:

1. Take a medium bowl, place all the ingredients in it, and stir well until combined.
2. Transfer the rub to an air-tight glass container and store until ready to use.

Nutrition:
Calories: 16, Carbs: 4 g, Fiber: 1 g, Sodium: 14 mg, Potassium: 49 mg, Phosphorus: 4 mg

6. Mixed Herb Blend
Preparation Time: 5 minutes
Cooking Time: 0 minutes
Servings: ⅓ cup, 2 tablespoons per serving
Ingredients:

- 1 tablespoon celery seed
- 2 tablespoons dried tarragon
- ¼ cup dried parsley
- 1 tablespoon dried oregano
- 1 tablespoon dill weed

Directions:

1. Take a medium bowl, place all the ingredients in it, and stir well until combined.
2. Transfer the rub to an air-tight glass container and store until ready to use.

Nutrition:
Calories: 20, Carbs: 4 g, Sodium: 9 mg, Potassium: 34 mg, Phosphorus: 7 mg

7. Poultry Seasoning
Preparation Time: 5 minutes
Cooking Time: 0 minutes
Servings: 11 teaspoons, 1 teaspoon per serving
Ingredients:

- 1 teaspoon ground black pepper
- 2 teaspoons dried marjoram
- 2 tablespoons dried ground sage
- 2 teaspoons dried thyme

Directions:

1. Take a medium bowl, place all the ingredients in it, and stir well until combined.
2. Transfer the rub to an air-tight glass container and store until ready to use.

Nutrition:
Calories: 3, Potassium: 8 mg, Phosphorus: 1 mg

8. Fajita Flavor Marinade
Preparation Time: 5 minutes
Cooking Time: 0 minutes
Servings: 1 cup
Ingredients:

- 1jalapeño pepper, finely diced
- 1 medium grapefruit, juiced
- ¼ teaspoon garlic powder
- 2 medium limes, juiced
- 3 tablespoons olive oil
- 1 medium orange, juiced

Directions:

1. Take a medium bowl, place all the ingredients in it, and stir well

until combined.

2. Pour the marinade over chicken or vegetables, toss until well coated, and let marinate for 1 hour.

3. Drizzle the marinade over chicken or vegetables and cook as instructed in the recipe.

Nutrition:
Calories: 33, Carbs: 2 g, Fat: 2.8 g, Fiber: 1 g, Potassium: 42 mg, Phosphorus: 5 mg

9. Garlic-Herb Seasoning
Preparation Time: 5 minutes
Cooking Time: 0 minutes
Servings: 1 ½ tablespoon, 1 tablespoon per serving
Ingredients:

- 2 teaspoons garlic powder
- 1 teaspoon powdered lemon rind
- 1 teaspoon dried oregano
- 1 teaspoon dried basil

Directions:

1. Add all the ingredients in the order in a food processor or blender and blend at medium speed until combined.

2. Tip the mixture in an air-tight glass container, add a few grains of rice to keep the mixture from clumping, and store until ready to use.

Nutrition:
Calories: 12, Carbs: 3 g, Fiber: 1 g, Sodium: 1 mg, Potassium: 47 mg, Phosphorus: 16 mg

10. Honey Mustard
Preparation Time: 5 minutes
Cooking Time: 0 minutes
Servings: 1 cup, 1 tablespoon per serving
Ingredients:

- ½ teaspoon onion powder
- 1 teaspoon garlic powder

- ¼ teaspoon ground white pepper
- 1 tablespoon ground mustard
- ¼ cup honey
- ¼ cup white vinegar
- ¾ cup olive oil

Directions:

1. Add all the ingredients in the order in a food processor or blender, except for oil and honey, and pulse at medium speed until blended.
2. Slowly blend in oil until incorporated and then mix in honey, 1 tablespoon at a time, until mustard reaches to desired sweetness.
3. Transfer the mustard into a bowl, then cover the bowl and store for up to 2 months in the refrigerator.
4. Serve when desired.

Nutrition:
Calories: 108, Carbs: 4.9 g, Fat: 10.2 g, Fiber: 0.3 g, Sodium: 0.5 mg, Potassium: 11.7 mg, Phosphorus: 25 mg,

11.   Soy Sauce
Preparation Time: 10 minutes
Cooking Time: 10 minutes
Servings: 3 tablespoons
Ingredients:

- ⅛ teaspoon garlic powder
- ⅛ teaspoon ground black pepper
- 2 teaspoons molasses
- 1 teaspoon apple cider vinegar
- 1 tablespoon red wine vinegar
- 2 tablespoons beef broth, reduced-sodium
- 1 teaspoon sesame oil
- ¼ cup water, hot

Directions:

1. Take a medium bowl, place all the ingredients in it, and stir

until combined.

2. Take a small saucepan, place it over medium-low heat, pour in soy sauce, and boil it until the sauce has reduced by half.

3. Then let the sauce cool completely, pour it into an air-tight glass container, cover with the lid, place it in the refrigerator and store for up to a month.

4. Serve when desired.

Nutrition:
Calories: 23, Carbs: 3 g, Fat: 1 g, Sodium: 25 mg, Potassium: 27 mg, Phosphorus: 6 mg

12. Barbecue Sauce
Preparation Time: 5 minutes
Cooking Time: 15 minutes
Servings: 1 cup, 1 tablespoon per serving
Ingredients:

- 6 oz. tomato paste, sodium-reduced
- 3 tablespoons water
- ¼ cup dark molasses
- ½ cup sautéed onion, minced
- ⅛ cup apple cider vinegar
- 2 tablespoons brown sugar
- 1 tablespoon Worcestershire sauce
- 1 tablespoon mustard
- 1 teaspoon lemon juice
- 1 ½ teaspoon BBQ rub for chicken

Directions:

1. Take a medium bowl, place all the ingredients in it, and stir until combined.

2. Take a small saucepan, place it over low heat, pour in barbecue sauce, and cook for 15 minutes.

3. Then let the sauce cool completely, pour it into an air-tight glass container, cover with the lid, and place it in the refrigerator, and store for up to two weeks.

4. Serve when desired.

Nutrition:
Calories: 34, Carbs: 8 g, Fiber: 2 g, Sodium: 53 mg, Potassium: 214 mg, Phosphorus: 2 mg

13.   Teriyaki Sauce
Preparation Time: 5 minutes
Cooking Time: 10 minutes
Servings: 1 cup, 1 tablespoon per serving
Ingredients:

- 1 ½ teaspoon minced garlic
- ½ cup brown sugar
- ¼ teaspoon ground ginger
- 2 tablespoons Chinese sweet rice wine
- 2 tablespoons sesame oil
- 1 cup soy sauce, sodium-reduced

Directions:

1. Take a small saucepan, place it over low heat, add all the ingredients in it, stir until just mixed, and cook for 5 to 10 minutes until the sugar has dissolved.
2. Then let the sauce cool completely, pour it into an air-tight glass container, cover with the lid, then keep it in the refrigerator and store for up to 1 month.
3. Serve when desired.

Nutrition:
Calories: 29, Carbs: 5 g, Protein: 1 g, Fiber: 1 g, Sodium: 308 mg, Potassium: 1 mg, Phosphorus: 308 mg

14.   Pizza Sauce
Preparation Time: 10 minutes
Cooking Time: 20 minutes
Servings: for a 12-inch pizza
Ingredients:

- 6 oz. tomato paste, sodium-reduced
- 2 tablespoons fresh basil
- 1 teaspoon dried oregano
- 2 tablespoons olive oil

- 1 teaspoon dried parsley
- 3 tablespoons water

Directions:

1. Take a medium bowl, add all the ingredients in it and stir until well mixed.
2. Pour the sauce into an air-tight glass container, cover with the lid, and store in the refrigerator for up to two weeks.
3. For serving, spread the sauce over a 12-inch pizza crust, then scatter with topping, and bake as instructed in the recipe.

Nutrition:
Calories: 68, Carbs: 9 g, Protein: 1 g, Fat: 3 g, Fiber: 3 g, Sodium: 131 mg, Potassium: 409 mg, Phosphorus: 2 mg

15.   Alfredo Sauce
Preparation Time: 5 minutes
Cooking Time: 15 minutes
Servings: 1 ¾ cup
Ingredients:

- 3 tablespoons all-purpose flour
- ½ teaspoon minced garlic
- ¼ teaspoon ground nutmeg
- ¼ cup olive oil
- 1 tablespoon lemon juice
- 2 cups of rice milk, unsweetened
- 4 oz. cream cheese, sodium-reduced
- ⅓ cup grated parmesan cheese, sodium-reduced

Directions:

1. Take a large skillet, place it over medium heat, add oil in it and when hot, add flour and whisk until well mixed.
2. Then stir in garlic and pour in milk, whisking continuously until smooth and bring the mixture to boil.
3. Continue cooking the sauce for 5 to 10 minutes until it has thickened to the desired consistency or reduced by half, then

stir in cream cheese until combined and remove the pan from heat.

4. Add remaining ingredients into the sauce, stir well until mixed, and let cool for 10 minutes.
5. Ladle sauce over broiled rice, steamed vegetables cooked chicken, etc., and serve.

Nutrition:
Calories: 173, Carbs: 9 g, Protein: 3 g, Fat: 14 g, Fiber: 2 g, Sodium: 142 mg, Potassium: 32 mg, Phosphorus: 75 mg

Breakfast Recipes

16.　Fine Morning Porridge
Preparation Time: 15 minutes
Cooking Time: 0 minutes
Servings: 2
Ingredients:

- 2 tablespoons coconut flour
- 2 tablespoons vanilla protein powder
- 3 tablespoons Golden Flaxseed meal
- 1 ½ cups almond milk, unsweetened
- Powdered erythritol

Directions:

1. Take a bowl and mix in flaxseed meal, protein powder, coconut flour, and mix well.
2. Add mix to the saucepan (placed over medium heat).
3. Add almond milk and stir, let the mixture thicken.
4. Add your desired amount of sweetener and serve.

Nutrition:
Calories: 259, Fat: 13g, Phosphorus: 30mg, Potassium: 124mg, Sodium: 31mg, Carbs: 5g, Protein: 16g.

17.　Hungarian's Porridge
Preparation Time: 10 minutes
Cooking Time: 5-10 minutes

Servings: 2
Ingredients:

- 1 tablespoon chia seeds
- 1 tablespoon ground flaxseed
- ⅓ cup coconut cream
- ½ cup of water
- 1 teaspoon vanilla extract
- 1 tablespoon almond butter

Directions:

1. Add chia seeds, coconut cream, flaxseed, water, and vanilla to a small pot.
2. Stir and let it sit for 5 minutes.
3. Add butter and place pot over low heat.
4. Keep stirring as butter melts.
5. Once the porridge is hot/not boiling, pour into a bowl.
6. Add a few berries or a dash of cream for extra flavor.

Nutrition:
Calories: 410, Fat: 38 g, Phosphorus: 30 mg, Potassium: 100 mg, Sodium: 11 mg, Carbs: 10 g, Protein: 6 g

18. Awesome Nut Porridge
Preparation Time: 10 minutes
Cooking Time: 15 minutes
Servings: 2
Ingredients:

- 1 cup cashew nuts, raw and unsalted
- 1 cup pecan, halved
- 2 tablespoons stevia
- 4 teaspoons coconut oil, melted
- 2 cups of water

Directions:

1. Chop the nuts in a food processor and form a smooth paste.

2. Add water, oil, stevia to the nut paste and transfer the mix to a saucepan.
3. Stir cook for 5 minutes on high heat.
4. Reduce heat to low and simmer for 10 minutes.
5. Serve warm and enjoy!

Nutrition:
Calories: 260, Fat: 22 g, Phosphorus: 15 mg, Potassium: 124 mg, Sodium: 30 mg, Carbs: 13 g, Protein: 6 g

19.   Super Scrambled Eggs
Preparation Time: 10minutes
Cooking Time: 10 minutes
Servings: 1
Ingredients:

- ½ cup cream cheese
- ¼ cup unsweetened almond or rice milk
- 3 eggs
- 2 egg whites
- 1 tablespoon finely chopped scallion, green part only
- 2 tablespoons unsalted butter
- 1 tablespoon chopped fresh tarragon
- Black pepper (ground), to taste

Directions:

1. In a mixing bowl, whisk eggs and whites. Add cream cheese, milk, scallions, and tarragon. Combine to mix well with each other.
2. Take a medium saucepan or skillet, add butter. Heat over medium heat.
3. Add egg mixture and stir-cook for 4-5 minutes until eggs are scrambled evenly.
4. Season with black pepper and serve warm.

Nutrition:
Calories: 238, Fat: 17 g, Phosphorus: 117 mg, Potassium: 152 mg, Sodium: 211 mg, Carbs: 3 g, Protein: 8 g

20.   Rhubarb Muffins

Preparation Time: 10 minutes
Cooking Time: 25 minutes
Servings: 2
Ingredients:

- ½ cup almond meal
- 2 tablespoons crystallized ginger
- ¼ cup of coconut sugar
- 1 tablespoon linseed meal
- ½ cup buckwheat flour
- ¼ cup brown rice flour
- 2 tablespoons powdered arrowroot
- 2 teaspoons gluten-free baking powder
- ½ teaspoon fresh grated ginger
- ½ teaspoon ground cinnamon
- 1 cup rhubarb, sliced
- 1 apple, cored, peeled, and chopped
- ⅓ cup almond milk, unsweetened
- ¼ cup olive oil
- 1 free-range egg
- 1 teaspoon vanilla extract

Directions:

1. In a bowl, mix the almond meal with the crystallized ginger, sugar, linseed meal, buckwheat flour, rice flour, arrowroot powder, grated ginger, baking powder, and cinnamon and stir.
2. In another bowl, mix the rhubarb with the apple, almond milk, oil, egg, and vanilla and stir well.
3. Combine the 2 mixtures, stir well, and divide into a lined muffin tray.
4. Place in the oven at 350°F and bake for 25 minutes.
5. Serve the muffins for breakfast.

Nutrition:
Calories 200, Fat: 4 g, Fiber: 6 g, Phosphorus: 30 mg, Potassium: 124 mg, Sodium: 20 mg, Carbs: 13 g, Protein: 8 g

21.   Buckwheat Granola
Preparation Time: 10 minutes

Cooking Time: 45 minutes
Servings: 1
Ingredients:

- 2 cups oats
- 1 cup buckwheat
- 1 cup sunflower seeds
- 1 cup pumpkin seeds
- 1½ cups dates, pitted and chopped
- 1 cup apple puree
- 6 tablespoons coconut oil
- 5 tablespoons cocoa powder
- 1 teaspoon fresh grated ginger

Directions:

1. In a large bowl, mix the oats with the buckwheat, sunflower seeds, pumpkin seeds, dates, apple puree, oil, cocoa powder, and ginger then stir well.
2. Spread on a lined baking sheet, press well, and place in the oven at 360°F for 45 minutes.
3. Leave the granola to cool down, slice, and serve for breakfast.

Nutrition:
Calories: 161, Fat: 3 g, Phosphorus: 36 mg, Potassium: 14 mg, Sodium: 31 mg, Fiber: 5 g, Carbs: 11 g, Protein: 7 g

22.   Mushroom Frittata
Preparation Time: 10 minutes
Cooking Time: 30 minutes
Servings: 1
Ingredients:

- ¼ cup coconut milk, unsweetened
- 6 eggs
- 1 yellow onion, chopped
- 4 oz. white mushrooms, sliced
- 2 tablespoons olive oil
- 2 cups baby spinach
- A pinch of salt and black pepper

Directions:

1. Heat a pan with the oil over medium-high heat, add the onion, stir and cook for 2-3 minutes.
2. Add the mushrooms, salt, and pepper, stir and cook for 2 minutes more.
3. In a bowl, mix the eggs with salt and pepper, stir well and pour over the mushrooms.
4. Add the spinach, mix a bit, place in the oven, and bake at 360°F for 25 minutes.
5. Slice the frittata and serve.

Nutrition:
Calories: 200, Fat: 3 g, Phosphorus: 30 mg, Potassium: 104 mg, Sodium: 13 mg, Fiber: 6 g, Carbs: 14 g, Protein: 6 g

23.   Breakfast Crepes
Preparation Time: 10 minutes
Cooking Time: 10 minutes
Servings: 1
Ingredients:

- 2 eggs
- 1 teaspoon vanilla extract
- ½ cup almond milk, unsweetened
- ½ cup of water
- 2 tablespoons agave nectar
- 1 cup coconut flour
- 3 tablespoons coconut oil, melted

Directions:

1. In a bowl, whisk the eggs with the vanilla extract, almond milk, water, and agave nectar.
2. Add the flour and 2 tablespoons oil gradually and stir until you obtain a smooth batter.
3. Heat a pan with the rest of the oil over medium heat, add some of the batter, spread it into the pan, and cook the crepe until it's golden on both sides then transfer to a plate.
4. Repeat with the rest of the batter and serve the crepes.

Nutrition:
Calories: 121, Fat: 3 g, Phosphorus: 20mg, Potassium: 94mg, Sodium: 32mg, Fiber: 6 g, Carbs: 14 g, Protein: 6 g

24.   Mushroom Tofu Breakfast
Preparation Time: 10 minutes
Cooking Time: 8-10 minutes
Servings: 2
Ingredients:

- 1 tablespoon of chopped shallots
- ½ cup of sliced white mushrooms
- ⅓ cup medium-firm tofu, crumbled
- ⅓ teaspoon turmeric
- 1 teaspoon of cumin
- ⅓ teaspoon of smoked paprika
- 3 tablespoons of vegetable oil
- Pinch garlic salt
- Pepper

Directions:

1. Take a medium saucepan or skillet, add oil. Heat over medium heat.
2. Add shallots, mushrooms, and stir-cook until they become softened for 3-4 minutes.
3. Add tofu, salt, spices, and stir-cook until tofu is tender and cooked well.
4. Serve warm.

Nutrition:
Calories: 217, Fat: 21 g, Phosphorus: 77 mg, Potassium: 147 mg, Sodium: 301 mg, Carbs: 3 g, Protein: 4 g

25.   Herbed Omelet
Preparation Time: 5 minutes
Cooking Time: 8-10 minutes
Servings: 2
Ingredients:

- 4 eggs

- 2 tablespoons water
- 1 ½ teaspoons vegetable oil
- 1 tablespoon chopped onion
- ¼ teaspoon basil
- ⅛ teaspoon tarragon
- ¼ teaspoon parsley (optional)

Directions:

1. Take a mixing bowl and beat eggs. Add water and spices, combine.
2. Take a medium saucepan or skillet, add oil. Heat over medium heat.
3. Add onion and stir-cook until become translucent and softened. Set aside.
4. Add the egg mixture to the pan and spread evenly.
5. Cook over both sides until well set and lightly brown.
6. Serve warm with cooked onions on top.

Nutrition:

Calories: 204, Fat: 14 g, Phosphorus: 201 mg, Potassium: 166 mg, Sodium: 174 mg, Carbs: 1 g, Protein: 14 g

26.   Cheesy Scrambled Eggs with Fresh Herbs
Preparation Time: 15 minutes
Cooking Time: 10 minutes
Servings: 4
Ingredients:

- 3 Eggs
- 2 Egg whites
- ½ cup Cream cheese
- ¼ cup Unsweetened rice milk
- 1 Tbsp. Chopped scallion, green part only
- 1 Tbsp. Chopped fresh tarragon
- 2 Tbsps. Unsalted butter
- Ground black pepper to taste

Directions:

1. In a bowl, whisk the eggs, egg whites, cream cheese, rice milk, scallions, and tarragon until mixed and smooth.
2. Melt the butter in a skillet.
3. Pour in the egg mixture and cook, stirring, for 5 minutes or until the eggs are thick and curds creamy.
4. Season with pepper and serve.

Nutrition:
Calories: 221, Fat: 19 g, Carbs: 3 g, Phosphorus: 119 mg, Potassium: 140 mg, Sodium: 193 mg, Protein: 8 g

27.   Turkey and Spinach Scramble on Melba Toast
Preparation Time: 2 minutes
Cooking Time: 15 minutes
Servings: 2
Ingredients:

- 1 tsp Extra virgin olive oil
- 1 cup raw spinach
- ½ clove Garlic, minced
- 1 tsp. grated Nutmeg
- 1 cup Cooked and diced turkey breast
- 4 slices Melba toast
- 1 tsp. Balsamic vinegar

Directions:

1. Heat a skillet over medium heat and add oil.
2. Add turkey and heat through for 6 to 8 minutes.
3. Add spinach, garlic, and nutmeg and stir-fry for 6 minutes more.
4. Plate up the Melba toast and top with spinach and turkey scramble.
5. Drizzle with balsamic vinegar and serve.

Nutrition:
Calories: 301, Fat: 19 g, Carbs: 12 g, Phosphorus: 215 mg, Potassium: 269 mg, Sodium: 360 mg, Protein: 19 g

28.   Vegetable Omelet
Preparation Time: 15 minutes

Cooking Time: 10 minutes
Servings: 3
Ingredients:

- 4 Egg whites
- 1 Egg
- 2 Tbsps. Chopped fresh parsley
- 2 Tbsps. Water
- Olive oil spray
- ½ cup Chopped and boiled red bell pepper
- ¼ cup Chopped scallion, both green and white parts
- Ground black pepper

Directions:

1. Whisk together the egg, egg whites, parsley, and water until well blended. Set aside.
2. Spray a skillet with olive oil spray and place over medium heat.
3. Sauté the peppers and scallion for 3 minutes or until softened.
4. Pour the egg mixture into the skillet over vegetables and cook, swirling the skillet, for 2 minutes or until the edges start to set. Cook until set.
5. Season with black pepper and serve.

Nutrition:

Calories: 77, Fat: 3 g, Carbs: 2 g, Phosphorus: 67 mg, Potassium: 194mg, Sodium: 229 mg, Protein: 12 g

29. Mexican Style Burritos
Preparation Time: 5 minutes
Cooking Time: 15 minutes
Servings: 2
Ingredients:

- 1 Tbsp. Olive oil
- 2 Corn tortillas
- ¼ cup Red onion, chopped
- ¼ cup Red bell peppers, chopped
- ½Red chili, deseeded and chopped
- 2 Eggs

- Juice of 1 lime
- 1 Tbsp. chopped Cilantro

Directions:

1. Turn the broiler to medium heat and place the tortillas underneath for 1 to 2 minutes on each side or until lightly toasted.
2. Remove and keep the broiler on.
3. Heat the oil in a skillet and sauté onion, chili, and bell peppers for 5 to 6 minutes or until soft.
4. Crack the eggs over the top of the onions and peppers and place the skillet under the broiler for 5 to 6 minutes or until the eggs are cooked.
5. Serve half the eggs and vegetables on top of each tortilla and sprinkle with cilantro and lime juice to serve.

Nutrition:
Calories: 202, Fat: 13 g, Carbs: 19 g, Phosphorus: 184 mg, Potassium: 233 mg, Sodium: 77 mg, Protein: 9 g

30.   Blueberry Muffins
Preparation Time: 15 minutes
Cooking Time: 30 minutes
Servings: 12
Ingredients:

- 2 cups Unsweetened rice milk
- 1 Tbsp. Apple cider vinegar
- 3 ½ cups All-purpose flour
- 1 cup Granulated sugar
- 1 Tbsp. Baking soda substitute
- 1 tsp. Ground cinnamon
- ½ tsp. Ground nutmeg
- Pinch ground ginger
- ½ cup Canola oil
- 2 Tbsps. Pure vanilla extract
- 2 ½ cups Fresh blueberries

Directions:

1. Preheat the oven to 375F.
2. Line the cups of a muffin pan with paper liners. Set aside.
3. In a small bowl, stir together the rice milk and vinegar. Set aside for 10 minutes.
4. In a large bowl, stir together the sugar, flour, baking soda, cinnamon, nutmeg, and ginger until well mixed.
5. Add the oil and vanilla to the milk mixture and stir to blend.
6. Add the milk mixture to the dry ingredients and stir until just combined.
7. Fold in the blueberries. Spoon the muffin batter evenly into the cups.
8. Bake the muffins for 25 to 30 minutes or until golden and a toothpick inserted comes out clean.
9. Cool for 15 minutes and serve.

Nutrition:
Calories: 331, Fat: 11 g, Carbs: 52 g, Phosphorus: 90 mg, Potassium: 89mg, Sodium: 35 mg, Protein: 6 g

31.   **Bulgur, Couscous, and Buckwheat Cereal**
Preparation Time: 10 minutes
Cooking Time: 25 minutes
Servings: 4
Ingredients:

- 2 ¼ cups Water
- 1 ¼ cups Vanilla rice milk
- 6 Tbsps. Uncooked bulgur
- 2 Tbsps. Uncooked whole buckwheat
- 1 cup Sliced apple
- 6 Tbsps. Plain uncooked couscous
- ½ tsp. Ground cinnamon

Directions:

1. In a saucepan, heat the water and milk over medium heat.
2. Bring to a boil, and add the bulgur, buckwheat, and apple.
3. Reduce the heat to low and simmer, occasionally stirring until the bulgur is tender, about 20 to 25 minutes.

4. Remove the saucepan from the heat and stir in the couscous and cinnamon.
5. Let the saucepan stand, covered, for 10 minutes.
6. Fluff the cereal with a fork before Servings.

Nutrition:
Calories: 159, Fat: 1 g, Carbs: 34 g, Phosphorus: 130 mg, Potassium: 116 mg, Sodium: 33 mg, Protein: 4 g

32.   Sweet Pancakes
Preparation Time: 10 minutes
Cooking Time: 5 minutes
Servings: 5
Ingredients:

- 1 cup all-purpose flour
- 1 Tbsp. Granulated sugar
- 2 tsps. Baking powder
- 2 Egg whites
- 1 cup Almond milk
- 2 Tbsps. Olive oil
- 1 Tbsp. Maple extract

Directions:

1. Mix the flour, sugar, and baking powder in a bowl.
2. Make a well in the center and place to one side.
3. In another bowl, mix the egg whites, milk, oil, and maple extract.
4. Add the egg mixture to the well and gently mix until a batter is formed.
5. Heat skillet over medium heat.
6. Add 1/5 of the batter to the pan and cook 2 minutes on each side or until the pancake is golden.
7. Repeat with the remaining batter and serve.

Nutrition:
Calories: 178, Fat: 6 g, Carbs: 25 g, Phosphorus: 116 mg, Potassium: 126 mg, Sodium: 297 mg, Protein: 6 g

33.   Breakfast Smoothie

Preparation Time: 15 minutes
Cooking Time: 0 minutes
Servings: 2
Ingredients:

- 1 cup frozen blueberries
- ½ cup Pineapple chunks
- ½ cup English cucumber
- ½ Apple
- ½ cup Water

Directions:

1. Put the pineapple, blueberries, cucumber, apple, and water in a blender and blend until thick and smooth.
2. Pour into 2 glasses and serve.

Nutrition:
Calories: 87, Carbs: 22 g, Phosphorus: 28 mg, Potassium: 192 mg, Sodium: 3 mg, Protein: 0.7 g

34.   Buckwheat and Grapefruit Porridge
Preparation Time: 5 minutes
Cooking Time: 20 minutes
Servings: 2
Ingredients:

- ½ cup Buckwheat
- ¼ Grapefruit, chopped
- 1 Tbsp. Honey
- 1 ½ cups Almond milk
- 2 cups Water

Directions:

1. Bring the water to a boil on the stove. Add the buckwheat and place the lid on the pan.
2. Lower heat slightly and simmer for 7 to 10 minutes, checking to ensure water does not dry out.

3. When most of the water is absorbed, remove, and set aside for 5 minutes.
4. Drain any excess water from the pan and stir in almond milk, heating through for 5 minutes.
5. Add the honey and grapefruit.

Nutrition:
Calories: 231, Fat: 4 g, Carbs: 43 g, Phosphorus: 165 mg, Potassium: 370 mg, Sodium: 135 mg

35. Egg and Veggie Muffins
Preparation Time: 15 minutes
Cooking Time: 20 minutes
Servings: 4
Ingredients:

- Cooking spray
- 4 Eggs
- 2 Tbsp. Unsweetened rice milk
- ½Sweet onion, chopped
- ½Red bell pepper, chopped
- Pinch red pepper flakes
- Pinch ground black pepper

Directions:

1. Preheat the oven to 350°F.
2. Spray 4 muffin pans with cooking spray. Set aside.
3. In a bowl, whisk together the milk, eggs, onion, red pepper, parsley, red pepper flakes, and black pepper until mixed.
4. Pour the egg mixture into prepared muffin pans.
5. Bake until the muffins are puffed and golden, about 18 to 20 minutes

Nutrition:
Calories: 84, Fat: 5 g, Carb: 3 g, Phosphorus: 110 mg, Potassium: 117 mg, Sodium: 75 mg, Protein: 7 g

36. Tasty Pancakes
Preparation Time: 15 minutes
Cooking Time: 12 minutes

Servings: 4
Ingredients:

- 1 cup all-purpose flour
- ½ cup sugar
- ½ teaspoon phosphorus-free baking powder
- 1 cup homemade rice milk
- 2 eggs
- 1 tablespoon unsalted butter

Directions:

1. Add the flour, sugar, and baking powder in a medium bowl. Stir well.
2. In a separate bowl, whisk together the rice milk and eggs.
3. Add the milk mixture to the flour mixture. Beat until incorporated.
4. Melt half of the butter in a pan over medium heat.
5. Scoop the batter, about ¼ cup for each pancake, into the pan.
6. Cook the pancakes part by part for about 3 minutes, until the edges are firm and the bottoms are golden.
7. Repeat with the remaining butter and batter.
8. Serve hot and enjoy!

Nutrition:

Calories 284, Fat: 6 g, Cholesterol: 114 mg, Carbs: 50 g, Sugar: 27 g, Fiber: 1 g, Protein: 7 g, Sodium: 40 mg, Calcium: 91 mg, Phosphorus: 114 mg, Potassium: 113 mg

37. Slow Cooked Oats
Preparation Time: 5 minutes
Cooking Time: 30 minutes
Servings: 6
Ingredients:

- 1 tablespoon non-dairy butter substitute
- 1 cup steel cut oats
- 2 cups non-dairy milk
- 1 cup water
- 2 teaspoons vanilla extract

- 1 tablespoon pure maple syrup
- ¼ cup and 2 tablespoons unsweetened peanut butter
- 1 ½ cups fresh blueberries

Directions:

1. Heat oil in a pan over medium heat.
2. Add the oats, stir frequently, and toast for 3 minutes.
3. Add the milk, water, and vanilla to boil increasing to medium-high heat.
4. Stir well.
5. Cover and cook for 20-30 minutes with low simmer heat.
6. Stir from time to time.
7. Add the maple syrup and peanut butter.
8. Stir to combine.
9. Place in Servings: bowls and decorate with blueberries.
10. Serve and enjoy!

Nutrition:
Calories: 242, Fat: 12 g, Carbs: 29 g, Sugar: 10 g, Fiber: 4 g, Protein: 7 g, Sodium: 112 mg, Calcium: 25 mg, Phosphorus: 59 mg, Potassium: 205 mg

38.   Brown Muffins
Preparation Time: 15 minutes
Cooking Time: 30 minutes
Servings: 18
Ingredients:

- Cooking spray
- ½ cup buckwheat flour
- ¾ cup almond flour
- 1 cup unbleached all-purpose flour
- 6 tablespoons cocoa powder
- 1 teaspoon baking powder
- ½ teaspoon of sea salt
- ½ cup light brown sugar
- ⅓ cup sunflower or other vegetable oil
- 2 large eggs
- 1 teaspoon pure vanilla extract
- ½ cup whole milk yogurt

- 2 large bananas, softened
- 4 large (6-ounce) Medjool dates, pitted, diced
- ⅓ cup roasted pumpkin seeds

Directions:

1. Preheat oven to 350°F.
2. Spray a muffin tray with cooking spray and set aside. Arrange for 18 muffins.
3. In a large bowl pour dry ingredients and whisk well. Set aside.
4. In a separate bowl beat with the electric mixer the sugar and oil until fluffy.
5. Add the eggs, one at a time beating until well included.
6. Add the vanilla, yogurt, and mashed banana. Stir until well incorporated.
7. Add slowly the dry components. Mix until combined well.
8. Add the diced dates and pumpkin seeds. Mix well.
9. Spoon into a muffin tray and bake for about 25 minutes.
10. Serve warm and enjoy!

Nutrition:

Calories: 185, Fat: 10 g, Cholesterol: 21 mg, Carbs: 25 g, Sugar: 13 g, Fiber: 3 g, Protein: 5 g, Sodium: 106 mg, Calcium: 54 mg, Phosphorus: 112 mg, Potassium: 249 mg

39.   Papaya Orange Smoothie
Preparation Time: 5 minutes
Cooking Time: 2 minutes
Servings: 1
Ingredients:

- 3-ounces papaya, cut in small pieces
- ½ cup unsweetened almond milk
- 1 teaspoon honey
- ½ teaspoon fresh ginger, grated
- 2 tablespoons lime juice
- 2 ice cubes

Directions:

1. Add the papaya, milk, honey, ginger, and lime to the blender.
2. Blend on medium speed for 15 seconds and add the ice cubes.
3. Blend on high speed for about 30 seconds until smooth.
4. Serve and enjoy!

Nutrition:
Calories: 85, Fat: 2 g, Carbs: 17 g, Sugar: 13 g, Fiber: 3 g, Protein: 1 g, Sodium: 94 mg, Calcium: 255 mg, Phosphorus: 25 mg, Potassium: 276 mg

40.   Easy Corn Pudding
Preparation Time: 10 minutes
Cooking Time: 40 minutes
Servings: 6
Ingredients:

- Unsalted butter, for greasing the baking dish
- 2 tablespoons all-purpose flour
- ½ teaspoon Ener-G baking soda substitute
- 3 eggs
- ¾ cup unsweetened rice milk, at room temperature
- 3 tablespoons unsalted butter, melted
- 2 tablespoons light sour cream
- 2 tablespoons granulated sugar
- 2 cups frozen corn kernels, thawed

Directions:

1. Preheat the oven to 350°F.
2. Greasing a baking dish with butter and set aside.
3. In a mixing bowl add the flour and baking soda substitute. Stir well and set aside.
4. In a separate bowl, whisk the eggs, rice milk, butter, sour cream, and sugar.
5. Stir the two mixtures until smooth.
6. Add the corn to the batter. Stir until well mixed.
7. Spoon the batter into the baking dish and bake for about 40 minutes.
8. Let the pudding cool for about 15 minutes.
9. Serve warm and enjoy!

Nutrition:
Calories: 182, Fat: 10 g, Cholesterol: 115 mg, Carbs: 23 g, Sugar: 2 g, Fiber: 6 g, Protein: 5 g, Sodium: 62 mg, Calcium: 58 mg, Phosphorus: 116 mg, Potassium: 198 mg

41.   Sliced Apple Cookies
Preparation Time: 5 minutes
Cooking Time: 0 minutes
Servings: 8
Ingredients:

- 1 large apple, cored
- 2 tablespoons almond butter
- ⅓ cup muesli
- ¼ cup fresh blueberries

Directions:

1. Slice apple horizontally into about 8 rings.
2. Sprawl some almond butter on every apple ring.
3. Sprinkle the muesli on top and add the blueberries.
4. Serve and enjoy!

Nutrition:
Calories: 134, Fat: 7 g, Carbs: 16 g, Sugar: 9 g, Fiber: 3 g, Protein: 4 g, Sodium: 4 mg, Calcium: 39 mg, Phosphorus: 92 mg, Potassium: 180 mg

42.   Chocolate & Banana Muffins
Preparation Time: 20 minutes
Cooking Time: 12 minutes
Servings: 12
Ingredients:

- 2 large, softened bananas
- 1 large egg
- ⅓ cup light brown sugar
- ¼ cup olive oil
- 2 tablespoons plain yogurt
- 1 teaspoon vanilla extract
- 1 cup unbleached, all-purpose flour
- ¼ teaspoon sea salt

- ½ teaspoon baking soda
- ¼ teaspoon nutmeg
- ⅓ cup almonds, sliced
- ⅔ cup dark chocolate chips

Directions:

1. Preheat the oven to 350°F.
2. Spray a muffin tray with cooking spray and set aside.
3. In a mixing bowl add bananas, egg, sugar, and oil and stir well.
4. Add yogurt and vanilla and mix with a fork until smooth.
5. Add the flour ¼ cup at a time, with salt and baking soda in between additions.
6. Stir well.
7. Combine almonds and chocolate chips.
8. Bake for about 12 minutes.
9. Serve and enjoy!

Nutrition:
Calories: 148, Fat: 7 g, Cholesterol: 15 mg, Carbs: 19 g, Sugar: 8 g, Fiber: 1 g, Protein: 3 g, Sodium: 111 mg, Calcium: 22 mg, Phosphorus: 45 mg, Potassium: 140 mg

43.   Savory Spring Muffins
Preparation Time: 10 minutes
Cooking Time: 30 minutes
Servings: 12
Ingredients:

- 1 tablespoon olive oil
- 1 cup red bell pepper, chopped
- 1 green bell pepper, chopped
- 1 cup onion, chopped
- 2 cup spinach, chopped
- 2 cloves of garlic
- 1 cup mushrooms, chopped
- 4 eggs

Directions:

1. Preheat oven to 350°F.
2. Heat oil in a pan.
3. Add peppers, onion and cook until tender.
4. Add spinach, garlic, and mushrooms and cook for 2 more minutes.
5. In a mixing bowl add the eggs and blend.
6. Stir in cooked vegetables.
7. Spread the batter into the muffin tray.
8. Bake for about 20 minutes.
9. Serve and enjoy!

Nutrition:
Calories: 54, Carbs: 3 g, Protein: 4 g, Sodium: 38 mg, Phosphorus: 57 mg, Potassium: 147 mg

Meat Recipes

44.   Quick Marinated Pork Fajitas
Preparation Time: 20 minutes
Cooking Time: 5 minutes
Servings: 4
Ingredients:

- 1 green bell pepper, sliced
- 1 medium onion, sliced
- 1lb lean, boneless pork, sliced into thin strips
- 2 tbsp. pineapple juice
- 4 flour tortillas, 8" size

What you need from the store cupboard:

- 2 garlic cloves, minced
- 1 tsp dried oregano
- ½ tsp cumin
- 2 tbsp. vinegar
- ¼ tsp hot pepper sauce
- 1 tbsp. canola oil

Directions:

1. Preheat oven to 325° F.
2. Place garlic, oregano, cumin, pineapple juice, vinegar, and hot sauce in a Ziploc bag.
3. Add pork strips and marinade for around 10 minutes.
4. Wrap tortillas in foil and heat in the oven as you fry the pork.
5. Heat a skillet and stir fry the pork and vegetables for 5 minutes.
6. Top the warm flour tortillas with the pork and vegetables and roll up.
7. Ideal served with guacamole, salsa, and sour cream.

Nutrition:
Calories: 274, Carbs: 19 g, Protein: 28 g, Potassium: 435 g, Phosphorous: 187 mg

45.   Italian Herb Rubbed Pork Fillet
Preparation Time: 2 hours
Cooking Time: 20 minutes
Servings: 4
Ingredients:

- 1 tbsp. Dijon mustard
- 1 14oz pork tenderloin

What you need from the store cupboard:

- 2 garlic cloves, minced
- 1 tsp dried rosemary
- 1 tsp dried thyme
- 1 tsp dried basil
- 1 tsp dried parsley
- 1 tsp black pepper
- 1 tbsp. vegetable oil

Directions:

1. Mix the spices with the mustard and garlic in a small bowl.
2. Rub the herb mixture over the pork tenderloin and chill for at least two hours.
3. Preheat oven to 400°F.

4. Heat the oil in a large skillet and brown the tenderloin on all sides.
5. Bake the pork for 20 minutes.

Nutrition:
Calories 178, Carbs: 1 g, Protein: 24 g, Potassium: 401 g, Phosphorous: 230 mg

46.   Balsamic Pork Chops with Cremini Mushrooms
Preparation Time: 30 minutes
Cooking Time: 20 minutes
Servings: 4
Ingredients:

- 1lb center-cut boneless pork chops, about 1" thick
- 4oz Cremini mushrooms
- 1 small onion
- 3 tbsp. balsamic vinegar
- 1 tsp unsalted butter

What you need from the store cupboard:

- ½ tsp dried rosemary
- ½ tsp dried thyme
- ¼ tsp black pepper
- ¼ tsp garlic powder
- 2 tbsp. canola oil

Directions:

1. Mix the balsamic vinegar with rosemary, thyme, pepper, and garlic powder.
2. Marinade the pork in the herb vinegar for 15 minutes.
3. Heat oil in a skillet and cook chops for around 6-8 minutes on each side. Set aside.
4. Add butter, mushrooms, and onions to the pan and sauté.
5. Serve the chops topped with onion and mushroom mixture.

Nutrition:

Calories 285, Carbs: 5 g, Protein: 28 g, Potassium: 560 g, Phosphorous: 274 mg

47.   Low Phosphorous Pulled Pork
Preparation Time: 10 minutes
Cooking Time: 1 hour 30 minutes
Servings: 16
Ingredients:

- 4lb boneless pork shoulder roast, cubed
- 1 cup onion, chopped
- 1 cup orange-flavored drink

What you need from the store cupboard:

- ½ cup ketchup, no salt added
- 3 tbsp. brown sugar
- 3 tbsp. red wine vinegar
- 2½ tbsp. Worcestershire sauce
- 1 tsp liquid smoke
- ½ tsp black pepper
- 3 cloves garlic, chopped
- 1 tbsp. oil

Directions:

1. Heat the oil in a skillet and fry the pork, onion, and garlic for 5 minutes.
2. Add all other ingredients and bring to a boil.
3. Simmer for at least one hour.
4. The pork is cooked when most of the liquid has evaporated and you can shred the pork with a fork.

Nutrition:
Calories 233, Carbs: 7 g, Protein: 22 g, Potassium: 365 g, Phosphorous: 197 mg

48.   Roast Rosemary & Oregano Lamb
Preparation Time: 10 minutes
Cooking Time: 1 hour 30 minutes
Servings: 16

Ingredients:

- 4 tbsp. butter
- 1 boneless leg lamb, well-trimmed, rolled, and tied (about 4-½ pounds)
- ¼ cup fresh rosemary leaves, chopped
- ¼ cup fresh lemon juice

What you need from the store cupboard:

- 2 garlic cloves
- 2 tbsp. oregano leaves, dried and crushed
- 1 tsp salt
- 1 tsp black pepper
- 1 cup water

Directions:

1. Preheat oven to 325°F.
2. Mix the oregano, rosemary, garlic, salt and pepper, and half the soft butter in a small bowl.
3. Make slits in the lamb and stuff with herb butter.
4. Coat the lamb with remaining herb butter.
5. Mix the remaining softened butter with lemon juice and pour over the lamb.
6. Cover with foil and bake for 30 minutes per pound.
7. Uncover for the last hour of cooking to allow the lamb to develop a crisp skin.

Nutrition:
Calories: 318, Protein: 30 g, Potassium: 394 mg, Phosphorous: 228 mg

49.   Chili Con Carne
Preparation Time: 10 minutes
Cooking Time: 2 hours
Servings: 4
Ingredients:

- ½ cup onion, chopped
- 1 stalk celery, chopped

- ½ cup green bell pepper, chopped
- 1½lb lean ground beef
- 1lb low-sodium stewed tomatoes

What you need from the store cupboard:

- 2 tbsp. chili powder
- 1½ cup water
- 1 tbsp. canola oil

Directions:

1. Heat oil in a large skillet on medium heat.
2. Fry, onion, celery, and bell pepper for 5 minutes.
3. Add beef and cook until brown.
4. Add tomatoes, chili powder, and water.
5. Bring to the boil then reduce the heat to low.
6. Simmer for at least 2 hours.
7. Serve with rice. If your daily potassium allowance will allow, then consider doubling the serving size.

Nutrition:

Calories: 132, Carbs: 5 g, Protein: 20 g, Potassium: 450 mg, Phosphorous: 180 mg

50.   Kidney-Safe Classic American Meatloaf
Preparation Time: 10 minutes
Cooking Time: 40 minutes
Servings: 6
Ingredients:

- 20 topping squares unsalted saltine-type crackers, crushed
- 2 tbsp. onion, finely chopped
- 1lb lean ground beef (10% fat)
- 1 large egg
- 2 tbsp. 1% low-fat milk

What you need from the store cupboard:

- ¼ tsp black pepper

- ⅓ cup catsup
- 1 tbsp. brown sugar
- ½ tsp apple cider vinegar
- 1 tsp water

Directions:

1. Preheat oven to 350° F.
2. Coat a loaf pan lightly with nonstick cooking spray.
3. Mix the crackers, onion, ground beef, egg, milk, and black pepper, together in a large bowl.
4. Press the mixture into the loaf pan and bake for 40 minutes.
5. While the loaf is cooking make the topping by mixing catsup, brown sugar, vinegar, and water in a small bowl.
6. Cover the meatloaf with the topping and bake for 10 more minutes. with sauce.
7. Slice into 6 portions and serve with potatoes and vegetables.

Nutrition:
Calories: 227, Carbs: 14 g, Protein: 13 g, Potassium: 255 mg, Phosphorous: 147 mg

51.   Beef Brisket
Preparation Time: 30 minutes
Cooking Time: 3 hours
Servings: 8
Ingredients:

- ½ medium onion, diced
- 1 stalk celery, diced
- 1 medium carrot, diced
- 1 tbsp. fresh parsley, diced
- 2½lb trimmed beef brisket (3-½ pounds untrimmed)

What you need from the store cupboard:

- 2 tsp black pepper
- 2 tbsp. canola oil
- 3 bay leaves
- 2 cup reduced-sodium beef broth

- 3 cup water
- 2 tbsp. balsamic vinegar

Directions:

1. Preheat oven to 350°F.
2. Sprinkle beef with pepper
3. Heat oil in a pan and brown the meat for 5 minutes on each side. Set beef aside.
4. Add the onion, carrot, and celery and cook for 5 minutes while deglazing the pan.
5. Add beef back to the pan with the bay leaves, parsley to vegetable mixture, broth, water, and balsamic vinegar.
6. Bring to the boil then cover and cook for 1½ hours.
7. Turn the meat and cook for a further 1½ hours or until the meat is tender enough to fork.
8. Remove the beef from the pan.
9. Use the vegetables to make a gravy and serve.

Nutrition:
Calories: 230, Carbs: 4 g, Protein: 29 g, Potassium: 346 mg, Phosphorous: 193 mg

52.   Reduced-Protein Beef Tibbs
Preparation Time: 10 minutes
Cooking Time: 40 minutes
Servings: 4
Ingredients:

- 1 medium onion, thinly sliced
- 1 medium tomato, chopped
- 1 medium green bell pepper, chopped
- 12oz lean stewing beef, cubed

What you need from the store cupboard:

- 2 tbsp. oil
- Salt and freshly ground black pepper

Directions:

1. Sauté the onion in a skillet until brown.
2. Add the beef and tomato and continue to cook.
3. Midway through cooking add the bell pepper.
4. Continue to cook until the meat is tender.
5. Season before serving.

Nutrition:
Calories: 220, Carbs: 5 g, Protein: 17 g, Potassium: 415 g, Phosphorous: 164 mg

53.   All American Burgers
Preparation Time: 10 minutes
Cooking Time: 20 minutes
Servings: 4
Ingredients:

- 3 tbsp. rice milk
- 5 salt-free soda crackers
- 1 large egg, beaten
- 1lb ground beef, 85% lean

What you need from the store cupboard:

- 1 tsp salt-free herb seasoning blend

Directions:

1. Combine the crackers with the milk in a bowl and leave to stand until soft.
2. Add the beaten egg to the crackers and then add the ground beef.
3. Shape the ground beef into patties.
4. Grill for around 8 minutes on each side.
5. Serve on a bun with salad and relish.

Nutrition:
Calories: 242, Carbs: 7 g, Protein: 22 g, Potassium: 328 g, Phosphorous: 188 mg

54.   Balsamic Pork Chops
Preparation Time: 10 minutes

Cooking Time: 20 minutes
Servings: 4
Ingredients:

- 4 pork chops, trimmed
- 3 tablespoons balsamic vinegar
- ½ teaspoon dried thyme
- ½ teaspoon dried rosemary
- ¼ teaspoon garlic powder
- ¼ teaspoon black pepper
- 2 tablespoons vegetable oil
- 1 teaspoon unsalted butter
- 4 oz. mushrooms, sliced
- 1 onion, sliced

Directions:

1. Coat pork chops with vinegar and season with herbs and spices.
2. Pour oil into a pan over medium heat.
3. Cook pork chops for 6 minutes.
4. Turn the pork chops and reduce heat.
5. Cover and cook for 10 minutes.
6. Transfer pork on a plate.
7. Add the butter, mushrooms, and onions.
8. Cook for 2 minutes.
9. Pour the onion and mushroom with cooking liquid on top of the pork chops before servings.

Nutrition:
Calories: 285, Protein: 28 g, Carbs: 5 g, Fat: 17 g, Cholesterol: 81 mg, Sodium: 79 mg, Potassium: 560 mg, Phosphorus: 274 mg, Calcium: 40 mg, Fiber: 0.7 g

55.   Braised Beef
Preparation Time: 20 minutes
Cooking Time: 1 hour and 30 minutes
Servings: 8
Ingredients:

- 2 lb. beef brisket, trimmed

- 2 teaspoons black pepper
- 2 tablespoons olive oil
- ½ onion, chopped
- 1 carrot, sliced
- 1 stalk celery, chopped
- 3 bay leaves, crumbled
- 1 tablespoon fresh parsley, chopped
- 2 cups low-sodium beef broth
- 3 cups water
- 2 tablespoons balsamic vinegar

Directions:

1. Preheat your oven to 350°F.
2. Season beef with black pepper.
3. Pour oil into a pot and brown the meat for 5 minutes per side.
4. Transfer meat to a plate and add onion, carrot, and celery.
5. Cook for 4 minutes.
6. Add bay leaves and parsley.
7. Put the meat on top of the veggies.
8. Add the rest of the ingredients.
9. Cover and bring to a boil.
10. Transfer contents of the pot to baking pan.
11. Bake in the oven for 1 hour.

Nutrition:
Calories: 230, Protein: 29 g, Carbs: 4 g, Fat: 11 g, Cholesterol: 84 mg, Sodium: 178 mg, Potassium: 346 mg, Phosphorus: 193 mg, Calcium: 30 mg, Fiber: 0.8 g

56. Herbed Pork Chops
Preparation Time: 15 minutes
Cooking Time: 15 minutes
Servings: 4
Ingredients:

- 4 pork chops
- 1 tablespoon fresh lime juice
- 1 tablespoon fresh cilantro, chopped
- ½ cup chives, chopped

- 2 green bell peppers, sliced into strips
- ⅛ teaspoon dried oregano leaves
- ¼ teaspoon ground black pepper
- 1 tablespoon butter, melted
- ¼ teaspoon ground cumin
- 1 tablespoon olive oil
- 1 lime

Directions:

1. Coat pork chops with lime juice.
2. Season with cilantro.
3. Mix the oregano, pepper, butter, and cumin.
4. Pour oil into a pan over medium heat.
5. Add the pork chops and cook for 4 minutes per side.
6. Add the oregano mixture and bell pepper.
7. Cook for 3 minutes.

Nutrition:

Calories: 265, Protein: 34 g, Carbs: 24 g, Fat: 15 g, Cholesterol: 86 mg, Sodium: 70 mg, Potassium: 564 mg, Phosphorus: 240 mg, Calcium: 22 mg, Fiber: 1.0 g

57.   Dijon Pork Chops
Preparation Time: 15 minutes
Cooking Time: 15 minutes
Servings: 4
Ingredients:

- 4 pork loin chops
- 2 tablespoons all-purpose flour
- ¼ cup shallots, chopped
- 2 teaspoons fresh ginger root, grated
- 1 tablespoon butter
- ½ cup low-sodium chicken broth
- 2 tablespoons dry sherry
- 2 teaspoons Dijon mustard
- 1 teaspoon mustard seed
- ⅛ teaspoon pepper
- Parsley

Directions:

1. Coat both sides of pork chops with flour.
2. In a pan over medium heat, add the butter and cook pork chops until golden brown.
3. Place on a platter and keep warm.
4. Add sherry and broth to the skillet.
5. Bring to a boil.
6. Lower heat.
7. Add the shallots and ginger root.
8. Cook for 2 minutes.
9. Add the rest of the ingredients.
10. Pour the sauce over the pork chops before serving.

Nutrition:

Calories: 296, Protein: 27 g, Carbs: 5 g, Fat: 17 g, Cholesterol: 78 mg, Sodium: 168 mg, Potassium: 438 mg, Phosphorus: 248 mg, Calcium: 34 mg, Fiber: 0.5 g

58.   Barbecue Beef
Preparation Time: 10 minutes
Cooking Time: 5 hours
Servings: 14
Ingredients:

- ¾ cup brown sugar
- 12 oz. beer
- 8 oz. ketchup
- 4 lb. chuck roast
- 14 hamburger buns

Directions:

1. Preheat your oven to 325°F.
2. Combine beer, brown sugar, and ketchup.
3. Add the roast to a baking pan.
4. Coat with the mixture.
5. Cover with foil.
6. Bake for 5 hours.
7. Slice meat or shred using a fork.

8. Serve on buns.

Nutrition:
Calories: 450, Protein: 33 g, Carbs: 32 g, Fat: 21 g, Cholesterol: 92 mg, Sodium: 261 mg, Potassium: 357 mg, Phosphorus: 207 mg, Calcium: 85 mg, Fiber: 0.6 g

59.   Pork Souvlaki
Preparation Time: 1 hour
Cooking Time: 15 minutes
Servings: 6
Ingredients:

- 3 tablespoons lemon juice
- ¼ cup olive oil
- ⅛ teaspoon black pepper
- 1 teaspoon dried oregano
- 1 lb. pork tenderloin, cubed
- 1 onion, sliced
- 2 cloves garlic, minced
- 1 bell green pepper, sliced

Directions:

1. In a bowl, combine lemon juice, oil, pepper, and oregano.
2. Marinate pork cubes in the mixture for 45 minutes inside the refrigerator.
3. Thread the pork, onion, and bell pepper into skewers.
4. Grill for 15 minutes, turning halfway through.
5. Serve with rice or salad.

Nutrition:
Calories: 204, Protein: 18 g, Carbs: 5 g, Fat: 13 g, Cholesterol: 53 mg, Sodium: 58 mg, Potassium: 336 mg, Phosphorus: 179 mg, Calcium: 17 mg

60.   Roasted Lamb
Preparation Time: 30 minutes
Cooking Time: 1 hour and 30 minutes
Servings: 10
Ingredients:

- ¼ cup fresh rosemary leaves
- 2 tablespoons dried oregano
- 1 teaspoon black pepper
- 2 garlic cloves, minced
- 4 tablespoons butter, divided
- 1 leg of lamb, trimmed
- ¼ cup fresh lemon juice
- 1 cup water

Directions:

1. Preheat your oven to 325°F.
2. In a bowl, combine the rosemary, oregano, pepper, and garlic.
3. Stir in 2 tablespoons butter.
4. Create slits on both sides of the lamb using a sharp knife.
5. Stuff these slits with herb and butter mixture.
6. Coat the lamb with the remaining mixture.
7. Cover with foil and bake for 1 hour.
8. Uncover the lamb and bake for another 30 minutes.

Nutrition:
Calories: 318, Protein: 30 g, Fat: 22 g, Cholesterol: 118 mg, Sodium: 114 mg, Potassium: 394 mg, Phosphorus: 228 mg, Calcium: 32 mg, Fiber: 0.5 g

61.   Italian Beef
Preparation Time: 30 minutes
Cooking Time: 5 hours and 45 minutes
Servings: 15
Ingredients:

- 3 lb. lean beef roast, trimmed
- 2 teaspoons oregano
- 2 teaspoons black pepper
- 1 teaspoon garlic powder
- 1 teaspoon red pepper, crushed
- 1 onion, sliced
- 1 green bell pepper, sliced
- 1 yellow bell pepper, sliced
- 1 red bell pepper, sliced
- ½ cup pepperoncini juice

Directions:

1. Put all the ingredients except the bell peppers, onion, and pepperoncini juice in a slow cooker.
2. Cook on high setting for 5 hours.
3. Shred beef and put it back in the pot.
4. Add the rest of the ingredients.
5. Cook on high setting for 45 minutes.

Nutrition:
Calories: 212, Protein: 25 g, Carbs: 3 g, Fat: 11 g, Cholesterol: 84 mg, Sodium: 121 mg, Potassium: 280 mg, Phosphorus: 196 mg, Calcium: 21 mg, Fiber: 0.6 g

62.　　Meat & Rice Balls
Preparation Time: 15 minutes
Cooking Time: 40 minutes
Servings: 4
Ingredients:

- 1 lb. lean ground beef
- 4 cups cooked white rice
- 1 egg
- ¾ teaspoon herb seasoning blend
- 2 ¼ cups water

Directions:

1. Mix the beef, rice and egg.
2. Roll and form 24 balls.
3. Cook the balls in a pan over medium heat.
4. Mix the herb seasoning and water.
5. Add the mixture to the pan.
6. Bring to a boil and then reduce heat and simmer covered for 30 minutes.

Nutrition:
Calories: 348, Protein: 24 g, Carbs: 18 g, Fat: 20 g, Cholesterol: 131 mg, Sodium: 95 mg, Potassium: 350 mg, Phosphorus: 197 mg, Calcium: 21 mg, Fiber: 0.5 g

63. Shish Kebabs
Preparation Time: 40 minutes
Cooking Time: 30 minutes
Servings: 6
Ingredients:

- ½ cup olive oil
- ½ cup white vinegar
- ¼ teaspoon garlic powder
- ½ teaspoon oregano
- ¼ teaspoon black pepper
- 1 ½ pounds' beef sirloin, cubed
- 2 onions, sliced
- 2 green bell peppers, sliced
- 1 red bell pepper, sliced

Directions:

1. Combine oil, vinegar, garlic powder, oregano, and pepper in a bowl.
2. Soak the beef cubes in the marinade for 30 minutes.
3. Thread beef cubes and vegetables into the skewers.
4. Grill for 30 minutes.

Nutrition:
Calories: 358, Protein: 26 g, Carbs: 5 g, Fat: 26 g, Cholesterol: 80 mg, Sodium: 60 mg, Potassium: 458 mg, Phosphorus: 217 mg, Calcium: 25 mg, Fiber: 1.4 g

64. Mongolian Beef Stew
Preparation Time: 10 minutes
Cooking Time: 14 minutes
Servings: 4
Ingredients:

- 2 lbs. flank steak, cut into thin strips
- ¼ cup cornstarch
- 1 cup of water
- ⅔ cup brown sugar
- 2 tablespoons rice vinegar

- 1 tablespoon sesame oil
- ½ teaspoons red pepper flakes
- 1 cup shredded carrots
- 4 cloves garlic, minced
- 2 teaspoons fresh ginger, minced
- 2 green onions, sliced
- 1 tablespoon sesame seeds to garnish

Directions:

1. Start by adding water, brown sugar, sesame oil, rice, and red pepper flakes.
2. Mix well then add carrots, sliced beef, ginger, and garlic.
3. Seal the lid and cook for 10 minutes on Manual Mode at High pressure.
4. Once the cooking is done, release the pressure completely then remove the lid.
5. Now mix ¼ cup water with cornstarch in a small bowl and whisk well.
6. Add this slurry to the beef and mix well.
7. Switch the Instant Pot to Sauté mode and cook for 4 minutes with occasional stirring.
8. Garnish with sesame seeds and green onion.
9. Serve warm.

Nutrition:

Calories: 275, Fats: 13 g, Cholesterol: 82 mg, Sodium: 122 mg, Carbs: 9 g, Fiber: 0.2 g, Sugar: 0.4 g, Protein: 26 g

65.   Chuck Beef Stew
Preparation Time: 10 minutes
Cooking Time: 31 minutes
Servings: 4
Ingredients:

- 1 ½ lb. beef chuck roast, diced
- ½ teaspoons black pepper
- 3 tablespoons olive oil
- 1 ½ cups red onion, diced
- 1 tablespoon minced garlic

- ¼ cup balsamic vinegar
- 2 cups carrots, diced
- 1 cup celery, diced
- 3 cups unsalted beef stock
- 2 tablespoons cornstarch
- ¼ cup water
- ¼ cup cilantro leaves
- ½ cup peas

Directions:

1. Start by mixing beef cubes with black pepper.
2. Heat 2 tablespoons of oil in the Instant Pot by selecting the Sauté mode.
3. Add beef cubes to the oil and sear for 2 minutes per side.
4. Transfer the beef cubes to a plate and keep them aside.
5. Add 1 tablespoon more oil to the Instant Pot along with onions.
6. Sauté for 1 minute, then add garlic to sauté for 30 seconds.
7. Stir in balsamic vinegar and deglaze the bottom by mixing for 3 minutes.
8. Toss in carrots, celery, beef cubes, stock.
9. Seal the lid and cook for 20 minutes on Manual mode at high pressure.
10. Once the cooking is done, release the pressure completely then remove the lid.
11. Mix cornstarch with water in a small bowl.
12. Pour this mixture into the pot and cook for 1 minute on Sauté mode.
13. Stir in peas and cook for 4 minutes.
14. Garnish with cilantro.
15. Serve warm.

Nutrition:

Calories: 343, Fats: 13 g, Cholesterol: 53 mg, Sodium: 281 mg, Carbs: 33 g, Fiber: 2.0 g, Sugar: 0.2 g, Protein: 24 g

66.   Taco Beef Barbacoa
Preparation Time: 10 minutes
Cooking Time: 49 minutes
Servings: 4

Ingredients:

- 2 tablespoons vegetable oil
- 2 lbs. beef stew meat
- 1 cup beef broth
- 2 tablespoons canned chipotle chiles in adobo sauce
- 3 cloves garlic, finely chopped
- 1 oz. sodium-free taco seasoning mix
- 1 teaspoon ground cumin
- 1 teaspoon ground coriander
- 2 cups red onions, chopped

Directions:

1. Start by heating oil in the Instant pot on sauté mode.
2. Add beef and sauté for 4 minutes per side until brown.
3. Stir in garlic, broth, chilies, taco seasoning, coriander, onion, and cumin.
4. Seal the lid and cook on Manual mode for 45 minutes on High pressure.
5. Once the cooking is done, release the pressure completely then remove the lid.
6. Shred the cooked beef and add ½ cup of the cooking liquid to it.
7. Serve warm.

Nutrition:
Calories: 210, Fats: 7 g, Cholesterol: 70 mg, Sodium: 85 mg, Carbs: 4 g, Fiber: 0.2 g, Sugar: 0.2 g, Protein: 28 g

67.   Pepperoncini Italian Beef
Preparation Time: 10 minutes
Cooking Time: 55 minutes
Servings: 8
Ingredients:

- 3 ½ lbs. boneless beef chuck, sliced
- 4 tablespoons unsalted butter
- 1 large red onion, peeled and sliced
- 6 cloves garlic, peeled and minced

- 20 pepperoncini peppers
- ¼ cup pepperoncini juices
- ½ cup Worcestershire sauce
- 1 cup beef broth
- 2 tablespoons brown sugar
- 1 tablespoon sodium-free dried Italian seasoning
- ½ teaspoons crushed red pepper

Directions:

1. Start by heating butter in an Instant Pot on Sauté mode.
2. Toss in garlic and onions, sauté for 5 minutes.
3. Stir in beef, pepperoncini's, Worcestershire sauce, Italian seasoning, red pepper, broth, sugar, and pepper juice.
4. Seal the lid and cook for 50 minutes on Manual Mode at High pressure.
5. Once the cooking is done, release the pressure completely then remove the pot's lid.
6. Shred the beef with a fork then serve.

Nutrition:
Calories: 267, Fats: 15 g, Cholesterol: 94 mg, Sodium: 176 mg, Carbs: 3 g, Fiber: 0.6 g, Sugar: 0.2 g, Protein: 30 g

68.   Hawaiian Pork
Preparation Time: 10 minutes
Cooking Time: 20 minutes
Servings: 2
Ingredients:

- 2 slices red onion
- 2 slices green bell pepper
- 2 boneless pork chops, 4 ounces each
- 4 canned pineapple slices
- 2 teaspoons teriyaki sauce
- 2 tablespoons trans-fat free margarine
- ⅛ teaspoon black pepper

Directions:

1. Toss the pork chops with black pepper, margarine, and sauce in a bowl.
2. Pour 1½ cups water in the Instant Pot and set the trivet over it.
3. Spread the chops in a baking dish and set the pineapple, onion, and bell pepper around the chops.
4. Seal the lid and cook for 20 minutes on Manual Mode at High pressure.
5. Once the cooking is done, release the pressure completely then remove the pot's lid.
6. Toss well and serve warm.

Nutrition:
Calories: 357, Fats: 17 g, Cholesterol: 69 mg, Sodium: 128 mg, Carbs: 28 g, Fiber: 1.5 g, Sugar: 0.9 g, Protein: 24 g

69.   Pork Roast with Vegetables
Preparation Time: 10 minutes
Cooking Time: 40 minutes
Servings: 4
Ingredients:

- 2 lbs. pork loin roast
- fresh cracked black pepper, to taste
- 2 tablespoons unsalted butter
- ½ medium onion, diced
- 4 cloves garlic, minced
- 2 medium carrots, chopped
- 2 stalks celery, chopped
- ½ cup broth or apple juice
- 2 Tablespoons Worcestershire sauce
- 1 Tablespoon brown sugar
- 1 teaspoon yellow mustard
- 2 teaspoons herbs of choice- dried or fresh
- 1 tablespoon corn starch
- ¼ cup water

Directions:

1. Start by seasoning the pork with black pepper.
2. Melt butter in an Instant pot on Sauté mode.

3. Add the pork and stir cook until golden brown.
4. Toss in garlic and onions, sauté for 2 minutes.
5. Stir in broth, celery, carrots, mustard, herbs, brown sugar, and Worcestershire sauce.
6. Mix well and seal the pot's lid.
7. Cook on Manual Mode for 30 minutes at high pressure.
8. Once the cooking is done, release the pressure completely then remove the pot's lid.
9. Allow the pork to rest for 10 minutes approximately.
10. Mix cornstarch with water in a bowl.
11. Pour this mixture into the pork and stir cook on Sauté mode until it thickens.
12. Serve.

Nutrition:
Calories: 294, Fats: 19.3 g, Cholesterol: 132 mg, Sodium: 76 mg, Carbs: 6.3 g, Fiber: 1.4 g, Sugar: 0.9 g, Protein: 45.1 g

70.   Beef Pot Roast
Preparation Time: 10 minutes
Cooking Time: 65 minutes
Servings: 6
Ingredients:

- 2-3 lbs. boneless beef chuck roast
- ½ teaspoons black pepper
- 2 tablespoons olive oil or butter
- 1 medium onion, sliced
- 4 cloves garlic, minced
- 1 cup chicken broth or beef broth
- 2 tablespoons yogurt
- 1 teaspoon dried herbs (thyme, oregano)
- 1 tablespoon Worcestershire sauce
- ½ cup red wine, optional
- 4 large carrots, cut into 1" cubes
- 3 stalks celery, chopped
- 8 oz. mushrooms, cut in half

Directions:

1. Start by seasoning the beef with black pepper.
2. Heat the olive oil in the Instant Pot on Sauté mode.
3. Stir in beef and sauté until it is brown.
4. Toss in garlic and onions, sauté for 5 minutes until soft.
5. Stir in yogurt, herbs, broth, beef, red wine, black pepper, and Worcestershire sauce.
6. Seal the lid and cook for 50 minutes on Manual Mode with High pressure.
7. Once the cooking is done, release the pressure completely then remove the pot's lid.
8. Remove the lid and add mushrooms, carrots, celery.
9. Seal the lid again and cook for another 10 minutes on Manual mode with High pressure.
10. Once the cooking is done, release the pressure completely then remove the pot's lid.
11. Serve warm.

Nutrition:

Calories: 343, Fat: 21.4 g, Cholesterol: 165 mg, Sodium: 45 mg, Carbs: 7.1 g, Fiber: 2.2 g, Sugar: 0.9 g, Protein: 33.4 g

Poultry Recipes

71.   Chicken with Vegetables and Worcestershire Sauce
Preparation Time: 15 minutes
Cooking Time: 3 hours
Servings: 2
Ingredients:

- 1 cup frozen sliced carrots
- 1 cup frozen green beans
- ½ cup diced onion
- 1-pound chicken breasts, boneless and skinless
- ½ cup low sodium chicken consommé
- 2 tsp. Worcestershire sauce
- 1 small spoon herb seasoning

Directions:

1. Put together carrots, green beans, and onion in a pan and cook them slowly.
2. Put the chicken breasts on vegetables and pour the consommé over the chicken.
3. Top with Worcestershire sauce and herb seasoning.
4. Cook at high heat for 3 hours or low heat for 6 hours.
5. Serve the chicken accompanied by the consommé in a cup and the vegetable mix. Enjoy!

Nutrition:
Calories: 180, Protein: 25 g, Sodium: 185 mg, Potassium: 430 mg, Phosphorus: 225 mg

72.   Chicken Meatballs
Preparation Time: 10 minutes
Cooking Time: 25 Minutes
Servings: 6
Ingredients:

- Red pepper flakes
- Pepper, to taste
- 1 tsp. minced garlic
- 1 egg
- 1 chopped scallion
- ¼ cup breadcrumbs
- ½ lb. ground chicken

Directions:

1. Turn your oven to 400°F.
2. Place red pepper flakes, pepper, garlic, egg, scallion, breadcrumbs, and ground chicken into a large bowl.
3. Mix everything using your hands.
4. Form this mixture into meatballs and put them on a baking sheet.
5. Allow them to cook for 25 minutes. Flip them over several times during cooking until they are golden brown. Serve and enjoy!

Nutrition: Calories: 85, Protein: 8 g, Sodium: 67 mg, Potassium: 200 mg, Phosphorus: 91 mg

73.   Chicken Salad Wraps
Preparation Time: 25 Minutes
Cooking Time: 0 minutes
Servings: 4
Ingredients:

- 4 large lettuce leaves
- Pepper, to taste
- ¼ cup mayonnaise
- 1 stalk chopped celery
- ½ cup seedless red grapes
- 1 chopped scallion
- 8 oz. cooked shredded chicken

Directions:

1. Place the mayonnaise, celery, grapes, scallion, and chicken into a bowl and mix well.
2. Sprinkle on some pepper and give another stir.
3. Take one lettuce leaf and spoon some chicken salad onto the middle.
4. Wrap the lettuce leaf around the chicken mixture. Serve and enjoy!

Nutrition:
Calories: 110, Protein: 13 g, Sodium: 61 mg, Potassium: 200 mg, Phosphorus: 117 mg

74.   Asian Style Pan-Fried Chicken
Preparation Time: 20 minutes
Cooking Time: 20 minutes
Servings: 4
Ingredients:

- 1 lemon, cut into wedges
- 3 tsp. canola oil, divided
- ½ cup cornstarch
- 1 tsp. low sodium soy sauce

- 1-inch piece minced ginger
- 1 tsp. dry rice wine
- 12 oz. chicken thighs, boneless and skinless

Directions:

1. Mix the soy sauce, ginger, rice wine, and chicken.
2. Toss everything together and allow it to marinate for 15 minutes.
3. Toss the chicken one more time and then drain off the liquid. One at a time, dip the chicken pieces into the cornstarch so that they are coated.
4. Heat 1½ teaspoons of oil on medium-high in a medium skillet.
5. Add half of the chicken to the skillet and cook until it has turned golden brown on one side, around 3 to 5 minutes. Turn the chicken over and continue to cook until the chicken has cooked through and browned. Place on a plate lined with a paper towel to cool and to absorb excess oil.
6. Add in the remaining oil and cook the rest of the chicken thighs.
7. Serve the chicken with a garnish of lemon. Enjoy!

Nutrition:
Calories: 198, Protein: 17 g, Sodium: 119 mg, Potassium: 218 mg, Phosphorus: 148 mg

75.   Curried Chicken with Cauliflower
Preparation Time: 2 hours 10 minutes
Cooking Time: 40 minutes
Servings: 6
Ingredients:

- Lime juice of 2 limes
- ½ tsp. dried oregano
- Cauliflower head, cut into florets
- 4 tsp. EVOO, divided
- 6 chicken thighs, bone-in
- ½ tsp. pepper, divided
- ¼ tsp. paprika
- ½ tsp. ground cumin

- 3 tbsp. curry powder

Directions:

1. Mix a quarter of a tsp. of pepper, paprika, cumin, and curry in a small bowl.
2. Add the chicken thighs to a medium bowl and drizzle with 2 tsp. olive oil and sprinkle in the curry mixture.
3. Toss them together so that the chicken is well coated.
4. Cover this up and refrigerate it for at least 2 hours.
5. Now set your oven to 400°F.
6. Toss the cauliflower, remaining oil, and oregano together in a medium bowl. Arrange the cauliflower and chicken across a baking sheet in one layer.
7. Allow this to bake for 40 minutes. Stir the cauliflower and flip the chicken once during the cooking time. The chicken should be browned, and the juices should run clear. The temperature of the chicken should reach 165.
8. Serve with some lime juice. Enjoy!

Nutrition:
Calories: 175, Protein: 16 g, Sodium: 77 mg, Potassium: 486 mg, Phosphorus: 152 mg

76.   Red and Green Grapes Chicken Salad with Curry
Preparation Time: 5 minutes
Cooking Time: 0 minutes
Servings: 2
Ingredients:

- 1 apple
- ¼ bowl seedless, red grapes
- ¼ bowl seedless, green grapes
- 4 cooked skinless and boneless chicken breasts
- 1-piece celery
- ½ bowl onion
- ½ bowl canned water chestnuts
- ½ tsp. curry powder
- ¾ cup mayonnaise
- ⅛ tsp. black pepper

Directions:

1. Cut the chicken into small dices and chop celery, onion, and apple. Drain and cut chestnuts.
2. Put together the chicken pieces, celery, onion, apple, grapes, water chestnuts, pepper, curry powder, and mayonnaise.
3. Serve it in a big salad bowl. Enjoy!

Nutrition:
Calories: 235, Protein: 13 g, Sodium: 160 mg, Potassium: 200 mg, Phosphorus: 115 mg

77. **Grilled Chicken Pizza**
Preparation Time: 5 minutes
Cooking Time: 12 minutes
Servings: 2
Ingredients:

- 2 pita bread
- 3 tbsp. low sodium BBQ sauce
- ¼ bowl red onion
- 4 oz. cooked chicken
- 2 tbsp. crumbled feta cheese
- ⅛ tsp. garlic powder

Directions:

1. Preheat oven at 350°F (that is 175°C).
2. Place 2 pitas on the pan after you have put non-stick cooking spray on it.
3. Spread BBQ sauce (2 tablespoons) on the pita.
4. Cut the onion and put it on pita. Cube chicken and put it on the pitas.
5. Put also both feta and the garlic powder over the pita.
6. Bake for 12 minutes. Serve and enjoy!

Nutrition:
Calories: 320, Protein: 22 g, Sodium: 520 mg, Potassium: 250 mg, Phosphorus: 220 mg

78. **Chicken Breast and Bok Choy**

Preparation Time: 15 minutes
Cooking Time: 20 Minutes
Servings: 4
Ingredients:

- 4 slices lemon
- Pepper, to taste
- 4 chicken breasts, boneless and skinless
- 1 tbsp. Dijon mustard
- 1 small leek, thinly sliced
- 2 julienned carrots
- 2 cups thinly sliced bok choy
- 1 tbsp. chopped thyme
- 1 tbsp. EVOO

Directions:

1. Start by setting your oven to 425°F.
2. Mix the thyme, olive oil, and mustard in a small bowl.
3. Take four 18-inch-long pieces of parchment paper and fold them in half. Cut them like you would make a heart. Open each of the pieces and lay them flat.
4. In each parchment piece, place ½ cup of bok choy, a few slices of leek, and a small handful of carrots.
5. Lay the chicken breast on top and season with some pepper.
6. Brush the chicken breasts with the marinade and top each one with a slice of lemon.
7. Fold the packets up and roll down the edges to seal the packages.
8. Allow them to cook for 20 minutes. Let them rest for 5 minutes, and make sure you open them carefully when serving. Enjoy!

Nutrition:
Calories: 164, Protein: 24 g, Sodium: 356 mg, Potassium: 189 mg, Phosphorus: 26 mg

79.   Baked Herbed Chicken
Preparation Time: 20 minutes
Cooking Time: 40 minutes

Servings: 6
Ingredients:

- ¼ tsp. pepper
- 6 chicken thighs, bone-in
- 1 tbsp. chopped oregano
- 1 tsp. lemon zest
- 1 tbsp. chopped parsley
- 4 garlic cloves, minced
- 4 tbsp. butter at room temperature

Directions:

1. Start by setting your oven to 425°F.
2. Add the lemon zest, parsley, oregano, garlic, and butter to a small bowl and mix well, making sure that everything is distributed evenly throughout the butter.
3. Lay the chicken on a baking pan and gently pull the skin back, but leaving it attached.
4. Brush the thigh meat with some of the butter mixture and lay the skin back over the meat. Sprinkle on some pepper.
5. Bake the chicken for 40 minutes. The skin should be crispy, and the juices should be clear. Also, the chicken should reach 165°F.
6. Allow the chicken to rest for 5 minutes before serving. Enjoy!

Nutrition:
Calories: 226, Protein: 16 g, Sodium: 120 mg, Potassium: 158 mg, Phosphorus: 114 mg

80.   Chicken and Cabbage Stir Fry
Preparation Time: 5 minutes
Cooking Time: 10 minutes
Servings: 4
Ingredients:

- Pepper, to taste
- ¼ cup water
- ½ tsp. garlic powder
- 1 tbsp. cornstarch
- 3 cups thinly sliced cabbage

- 1 tsp. ground ginger
- 10 oz. thinly sliced boneless, skinless chicken breast
- 1 tsp. canola oil

Directions:

1. Add the oil to a large skillet and heat. Add in the chicken and cook well, stirring often until it is cooked through and browned.
2. Add the cabbage into the skillet and cook for another 2 to 3 minutes. The cabbage should become tender, but it should still be green and crisp.
3. In a separate bowl, combine the water, garlic, ginger, and cornstarch. Pour this into the skillet and cook everything until the sauce has thickened up about 1 minute.
4. Season with some pepper. Serve and enjoy!

Nutrition:
Calories: 96, Protein: 15 g, Sodium: 156 mg, Potassium: 140 mg, Phosphorus: 15 mg

81. Chicken Meatloaf with Veggies
Preparation Time: 20 minutes
Cooking Time: 1-1¼ hours
Servings: 4
Ingredients:
For the meatloaf:

- ½ cup of cooked chickpeas
- 2 egg whites
- 2½ teaspoons of poultry seasoning
- Salt and freshly ground black pepper, to taste
- 10-ounce lean ground chicken
- 1 cup of red bell pepper (seeded and minced)
- 1 cup of the celery stalk (minced)
- ⅓ cup of steel-cut oats
- 1 cup of tomato puree (divided)
- 2 tablespoons of dried onion flakes (crushed)
- 1 tablespoon of prepared mustard

For the veggies:

- 2 pounds of summer squash (sliced)
- 16-ounce of frozen Brussels sprouts
- 2 tablespoons of extra-virgin olive oil
- Salt and freshly ground black pepper, to taste

Directions:

1. Preheat the oven to 350°F. Grease a 9x5-inch loaf pan.
2. In a mixer, add chickpeas, egg whites, poultry seasoning, salt, and black pepper. Then, pulse till smooth.
3. Transfer a combination in a large bowl.
4. Add chicken, veggies oats, ½ cup of tomato puree, and onion flakes. Then, mix till well combined.
5. Transfer the amalgamation into the prepared loaf pan evenly.
6. With both hands, press, down the amalgamation slightly.
7. In another bowl, mix mustard and the remaining tomato puree.
8. Place the mustard mixture over the loaf pan evenly.
9. Bake approximately 1-1¼ hours or till the desired doneness.
10. Meanwhile, in a big pan of water, arrange a steamer basket.
11. Bring to a boil and set summer squash in a steamer basket.
12. Cover and steam for approximately 10 to 12 minutes.
13. Drain well and aside.
14. Now, prepare the Brussels sprouts according to the package's directions.
15. In a big bowl, add veggies, oil, salt, and black pepper. Then, toss to coat well.
16. Serve the meatloaf with veggies.

Nutrition:
Calories: 420, Fat: 9 g, Carbs: 21 g, Fiber: 14 g, Protein: 36 g, Phosphorus: 431 mg, Potassium: 472 mg, Sodium: 249 mg

82. Turkey Pinwheels
Preparation Time: 10 minutes
Cooking Time: 15 minutes
Servings: 6
Ingredients:

- 6 toothpicks
- 8 oz. of spring mix salad greens
- 1 ten-inch tortilla
- 2 ounces of thinly sliced deli turkey
- 9 teaspoons. of whipped cream cheese
- 1 roasted red bell pepper

Directions:

1. Cut the red bell pepper into ten strips about a quarter-inch thick.
2. Spread the whipped cream cheese on the tortilla evenly.
3. Add the salad greens to create a base layer, then lay the turkey on top of it.
4. Space out the red bell pepper strips on top of the turkey.
5. Tuck the end and begin rolling the tortilla inward.
6. Use toothpicks to hold the roll into place and cut it into six pieces.
7. Serve with the swirl facing upward.

Nutrition:
Calories: 206, Fat: 9 g, Carbs: 21 g, Protein: 9 g, Sodium: 533 mg, Potassium: 145 mg, Phosphorus: 47 mg

83.   Chicken Tacos
Preparation Time: 5 minutes
Cooking Time: 20 minutes
Servings: 4
Ingredients:

- 8 corn tortillas
- 1½ teaspoon. of Sodium-free taco seasoning
- 1 juiced lime
- ½ cups of cilantro
- 2 green onions, chopped
- 8 oz. of iceberg or romaine lettuce, shredded or chopped
- ¼ cup of sour cream
- 1 pound of boneless and skinless chicken breast

Directions:

1. Cook chicken by boiling for twenty minutes.
2. Shred or chop cooked chicken into fine bite-sized pieces.
3. Mix the seasoning and lime juice with the chicken.
4. Put chicken mixture and lettuce in tortillas.
5. Top with green onions, cilantro, and sour cream.

Nutrition:
Calories: 260, Fat: 3 g, Carbs: 36 g, Protein: 23 g, Sodium: 922 mg, Potassium: 445 mg, Phosphorus: 357 mg

84.   Carrot & Ginger Chicken Noodles
Preparation Time: 5 minutes
Cooking Time: 10 minutes
Servings: 4
Ingredients:

- 1 sliced green onion
- 2 teaspoons. of grated fresh ginger
- 4 oz. skinless sliced chicken breasts
- 1 lime
- 1 minced garlic clove
- 1 cup of cooked rice noodles
- 1 teaspoon. coconut oil
- 1 peeled and grated carrot

Directions:

1. Heat a large pan over medium to high heat.
2. Add the coconut oil to a pan, and once melted, add the sliced chicken and brown for 4 to 5 minutes.
3. Now, add the ginger and garlic and sauté for 4 to 5 minutes.
4. Add green onion, carrot, and lime juice to the wok.
5. Put the cooked noodles into the pan and toss until hot through.
6. Serve hot and enjoy.

Nutrition:
Calories: 187, Protein: 11 g, Carbs: 25 g, Fat: 5 g, Sodium: 39 mg, Potassium: 91 mg, Phosphorus: 178 mg

85.   Lemon & Herb Chicken Wraps
Preparation Time: 5 minutes

Cooking Time: 30 minutes
Servings: 4
Ingredients:

- 4 oz. skinless and sliced chicken breasts
- ½ sliced red bell pepper
- 1 lemon
- 4 large iceberg lettuce leaves
- 1 tablespoon. of olive oil
- 2 tablespoons of finely chopped fresh cilantro
- ¼ teaspoon. of black pepper

Directions:

1. Preheat the oven to 375°F.
2. Mix the oil, juice of ½ lemon, cilantro, and black pepper.
3. Marinate the chicken in the oil marinade, cover, and leave in the fridge for as long as possible.
4. Wrap the chicken in parchment paper, drizzling over the remaining marinade.
5. Place in the oven in an oven dish for 25-30 minutes, or until chicken is thoroughly cooked through, and white inside.
6. Divide the sliced bell pepper and layer it onto each lettuce leaf.
7. Divide the chicken onto each lettuce leaf, and squeeze over the remaining lemon juice to taste.
8. Wrap and enjoy.

Nutrition:
Calories: 364, Protein: 35 g, Carbs: 32 g, Fat: 10 g, Sodium: 398 mg, Potassium: 413 mg, Phosphorus: 264 mg

86.   Turkey Sausages
Preparation Time: 10 minutes
Cooking Time: 10 minutes
Servings: 2
Ingredients:

- ¼ teaspoon of salt
- ⅛ teaspoon of garlic powder
- ⅛ teaspoon of onion powder

- 1 teaspoon of fennel seed
- 1 pound of 7% fat ground turkey

Directions:

1. Press the fennel seed.
2. In a small cup put together turkey with fennel seed, garlic, onion powder, and salt.
3. Cover the bowl and refrigerate overnight.
4. Prepare the turkey with seasoning into different portions with a circle form and press them into patties ready to be cooked.
5. Cook at medium heat until browned.
6. Cook it for 1 to 2 minutes per side and serve them hot. Enjoy!

Nutrition:
Calories: 55, Protein: 7 g, Sodium: 70 mg, Potassium: 105 mg, Phosphorus: 75 mg

87.   Rosemary Chicken
Preparation Time: 10 minutes
Cooking Time: 10 minutes
Servings: 2
Ingredients:

- 2 zucchinis
- 1 carrot
- 1 teaspoon of dried rosemary
- 4 chicken breasts
- ½ bell pepper
- ½ red onion
- 8 garlic cloves
- Olive oil
- ¼ tablespoon of ground pepper

Directions:

1. Prepare the oven and preheat it at 375°F (or 200°C).
2. Slice both zucchini and carrots. Then, add bell pepper, onion, and garlic.
3. Put everything in a 13" x 9" pan and add oil.

4. Spread the pepper over everything, and roast for about 10 minutes.
5. Meanwhile, lift the chicken skin, and spread black pepper and rosemary on the flesh.
6. Remove the vegetable pan from the oven and add the chicken, returning the pan to the oven for about 30 more minutes.
7. Serve and enjoy!

Nutrition:
Calories: 215, Protein: 28 g, Sodium: 105 mg, Potassium: 580 mg, Phosphorus: 250 mg

88.   Smoky Turkey Chili
Preparation Time: 5 minutes
Cooking Time: 45 minutes
Servings: 8
Ingredients:

- 12ounce lean ground turkey
- ½ red onion (chopped)
- 2 cloves of garlic (crushed and chopped)
- ½ teaspoon of smoked paprika
- ½ teaspoon of chili powder
- ½ teaspoon of dried thyme
- ¼ cup of low-sodium beef stock
- ½ cup of water
- 1 ½ cups of baby spinach leaves, washed
- 3 wheat tortillas

Directions:

1. Brown the ground beef in a dry skillet over medium-high heat.
2. Add in the red onion and garlic.
3. Sauté the onion until it goes clear.
4. Transfer the contents of the skillet to the slow cooker.
5. Add the remaining ingredients and simmer on Low for 30 to 45 minutes.
6. Stir through the spinach for the last few minutes to wilt.
7. Slice tortillas and gently toast under the broiler until slightly crispy.

8. Serve on top of the turkey chili.

Nutrition:
Calories: 93.5, Protein: 8g, Carbs: 3g, Fat: 5.5g, Cholesterol: 30.5mg, Sodium: 84.5mg, Potassium: 142.5mg, Phosphorus: 92.5mg, Calcium: 29mg, Fiber: 0.5g

89.   Avocado-Orange Grilled Chicken
Preparation Time: 20 minutes
Cooking Time: 60 minutes
Servings: 4
Ingredients:

- ¼ cup of fresh lime juice
- ¼ cup of minced red onion
- 1 avocado
- 1 cup of low-fat yogurt
- 1 small red onion, sliced thinly
- 1 tablespoon of honey
- 2 oranges, peeled and sectioned
- 2 tablespoons of chopped cilantro
- 4 pieces of 4-6ounce boneless, skinless chicken breasts
- Pepper and salt to taste

Directions:

1. Mix honey, cilantro, minced red onion, and yogurt in a large bowl.
2. Submerge chicken into mixture and marinate for at least 30 minutes.
3. Grease grate and preheat grill to medium-high fire.
4. Remove chicken from marinade and season with pepper and salt.
5. Grill for 6 minutes per side, or until chicken is cooked and juices run clear.
6. Meanwhile, peel the avocado and discard the seed. Then, chop and place in a bowl.
7. Quickly add lime juice and toss avocado to coat well with juice.
8. Add cilantro, thinly sliced onions, and oranges into a bowl of avocado, and mix well.

9. Serve grilled chicken and avocado dressing on the side.

Nutrition:
Calories: 209, Carbs: 26 g, Protein: 8 g, Fats: 10 g, Phosphorus: 157 mg, Potassium: 548 mg, Sodium: 125 mg

90.   Ciabatta Rolls with Chicken Pesto
Preparation Time: 10 minutes
Cooking Time: 20 minutes
Servings: 2
Ingredients:

- 6 teaspoons. of Greek yogurt
- 6 teaspoons. of pesto
- 2 small ciabatta rolls
- 8 oz. of a shredded iceberg or romaine lettuce
- 8 oz. of cooked boneless and skinless chicken breast (shredded)
- .125 teaspoons. of pepper

Directions:

1. Combine the shredded chicken, pesto, pepper, and Greek yogurt in a medium-sized bowl.
2. Slice and toast the ciabatta rolls.
3. Divide the shredded chicken and pesto mixture in half and make sandwiches with the ciabatta rolls.
4. Top with shredded lettuce if desired.

Nutrition:
Calories: 374, Fat: 10 g, Carbs: 40 g, Protein: 30 g, Sodium: 522 mg, Potassium: 360 mg, Phosphorus: 84 mg

91.   Grilled Spiced Turkey
Preparation Time: 5 minutes
Cooking Time: 20 minutes
Servings: 4
Ingredients:

- 6 oz. skinless and sliced turkey breast
- 1 tsp. cinnamon
- 1 tsp. curry powder

- 1 tbsp. olive oil
- 1 tsp. nutmeg

Directions:

1. Whisk the oil and spices together and baste the turkey slices, coating thoroughly.
2. Cover and leave to marinate for as long as possible (ideally overnight).
3. When ready to cook, preheat the broiler to medium-high heat and layer the turkey slices on a baking tray.
4. Place under the broiler for 15-20 minutes or according to package directions.
5. Turn occasionally.

Nutrition:
Calories: 101, Protein: 9 g, Carbs: 6 g, Fat: 11 g, Sodium: 42 mg, Potassium: 27 mg, Phosphorus: 102 mg

92.   Herb Chicken Stew
Preparation Time: 5 minutes
Cooking Time: 40 minutes
Servings: 6
Ingredients:

- 10 oz. skinless and diced chicken breast
- ½ cup white rice
- ½ diced red onion
- 1 tsp. dried oregano
- 1 tsp. dried thyme
- 1 tsp. olive oil
- ½ cup diced eggplant
- Black pepper
- 1 cup water

Directions:

1. Soak vegetables in warm water before use if possible.
2. Heat an oven-proof pot over medium-high heat and add olive oil.

3. Add the diced chicken breast and brown in the pot for 5-6 minutes, stirring to brown each side.
4. Once the chicken is browned, lower the heat to medium and add the vegetables to the pot to sauté for 5-6 minutes - careful not to let the vegetable brown.
5. Add the water, herbs, and pepper and bring to the boil.
6. Reduce the heat and simmer (lid on) for 30-40 minutes or until the chicken is thoroughly cooked through.
7. Meanwhile, prepare your rice by rinsing in cold water first and then adding to a pan of cold water and bringing to a boil over high heat.
8. Reduce the heat to medium and cook for 15 minutes.
9. Drain the rice and add it back to the pan with the lid on to steam until the stew is ready.
10. Serve the stew on a bed of rice and enjoy!

Nutrition:
Calories: 143, Protein: 15 g, Carbs: 9 g, Fat: 5 g, Sodium: 12 mg, Potassium: 20 mg, Phosphorus: 153 mg

93.   Lemon & Herb Chicken Wraps
Preparation Time: 5 minutes
Cooking Time: 30 minutes
Servings: 4
Ingredients:

- 4 oz. skinless and sliced chicken breasts
- ½ sliced red bell pepper
- 1 lemon
- 4 large iceberg lettuce leaves
- 1 tbsp. olive oil
- 2 tbsps. Finely chopped fresh cilantro
- ¼ tsp. black pepper

Directions:

1. Preheat the oven to 375°F/Gas Mark 5.
2. Mix the oil, juice of ½ lemon, cilantro, and black pepper.
3. Marinate the chicken in the oil marinade, cover, and leave in the fridge for as long as possible.

4. Wrap the chicken in parchment paper, drizzling over the remaining marinade.
5. Place in the oven in an oven dish for 25-30 minutes or until chicken is thoroughly cooked through and white inside.
6. Divide the sliced bell pepper and layer it onto each lettuce leaf.
7. Divide the chicken onto each lettuce leaf and squeeze over the remaining lemon juice to taste.
8. Season with a little extra black pepper if desired.
9. Wrap and enjoy!

Nutrition:
Calories: 200, Protein: 9 g, Carbs: 5 g, Fat: 13 g, Sodium: 25 mg, Potassium: 125 mg, Phosphorus: 81 mg

94.   Carrot & Ginger Chicken Noodles
Preparation Time: 5 minutes
Cooking Time: 10 minutes
Servings: 4
Ingredients:

- 1 sliced green onion
- 2 tsps. grated fresh ginger
- 4 oz. skinless sliced chicken breasts
- 1 lime
- 1 minced garlic clove
- 1 cup cooked rice noodles
- 1 tsp. coconut oil
- 1 peeled and grated carrot

Directions:

1. Heat a wok or large pan over medium-high heat.
2. Add the coconut oil to a pan and once melted, add the sliced chicken and brown for 4-5 minutes.
3. Now add the ginger and garlic and sauté for 4-5 minutes.
4. Add the green onion, carrot, and lime juice to the wok.
5. Add the cooked noodles to the wok and toss until hot through.
6. Serve piping hot and enjoy.

Nutrition:

Calories: 187, Protein: 11 g, Carbs: 25 g, Fat: 5 g, Sodium: 39 mg, Potassium: 91 mg, Phosphorus: 178 mg

95.   Chicken Kebab Sandwich
Preparation Time: 15 minutes
Cooking Time: 15 minutes
Servings: 4
Ingredients:

- 12 ounces boneless, skinless chicken breast
- 2 tablespoons freshly squeezed lemon juice
- 1 tablespoon extra-virgin olive oil
- 4 garlic cloves, minced, divided
- Freshly ground black pepper
- ¼ cup plain, unsweetened yogurt
- 4 white flatbreads
- 1 cucumber, sliced
- 1 cup lettuce, shredded

Directions:

1. In a medium bowl, add the chicken breast, lemon juice, olive oil, and half the garlic, tossing to coat. Season with pepper. Set aside to marinate while you prepare the other ingredients.
2. In a small bowl, add the yogurt and remaining garlic. Season with pepper and mix well. Set aside.
3. Heat a large skillet over medium-high heat and add the chicken and the marinade. Cook for 5 minutes, until the chicken, is well browned on the underside. Flip it over and cook the other side until the chicken is golden brown and the juices run clear. Remove from the pan and let rest for 5 minutes. Cut the chicken into thin slices.
4. In each flatbread, add some chicken, cucumber, and lettuce. Top with the yogurt sauce and serve.

Nutrition:
Calories: 217, Fat: 6 g, Cholesterol: 49 mg, Carbs: 21 g, Fiber: 1 g, Protein: 22 g, Phosphorus: 80 mg, Potassium: 231 mg, Sodium: 339 mg

96.   Aromatic Chicken and Cabbage Stir-Fry
Preparation Time: 10 minutes

Cooking Time: 10 minutes
Servings: 4
Ingredients:

- 1 teaspoon canola oil
- 10 ounces boneless, skinless chicken breast, thinly sliced
- 3 cups green cabbage, thinly sliced
- 1 tablespoon cornstarch
- 1 teaspoon ground ginger
- ½ teaspoon garlic powder
- ¼ cup water
- Freshly ground black pepper

Directions:

1. In a large skillet over medium-high heat, heat the oil. Add the chicken and cook, stirring often, until browned and cooked through.
2. Add the cabbage to the pan, and cook for another 2 to 3 minutes, until the cabbage is tender but still crisp and green.
3. In a small bowl, mix the cornstarch, ginger, garlic, and water. Add the mixture to the pan, and continue cooking until the sauce has slightly thickened about 1 minute. Season with pepper.

Nutrition:
Calories: 96, Fat: 2 g, Cholesterol: 38 mg, Carbs: 5 g, Fiber: 1 g, Protein: 15 g, Phosphorus: 15 mg, Potassium: 140 mg, Sodium: 156 mg

97.   Chicken Chow Mein
Preparation Time: 10 minutes
Cooking Time: 15 minutes
Servings: 6
Ingredients:

- 2 teaspoons cornstarch
- 1 tablespoon water
- 1 teaspoon low-sodium soy sauce
- 1 teaspoon of rice wine
- 1 teaspoon sugar

- 1 teaspoon sesame oil
- 2 teaspoons canola oil
- 3 garlic cloves, minced
- 8 ounces boneless, skinless chicken thighs, thinly sliced
- 2 cups shredded green cabbage
- 1 carrot, julienned
- 4 scallions, cut into 2-inch pieces
- 10 oz. chow mein noodles, cooked according to package directions
- 1 cup mung bean sprouts

Directions:

1. In a small bowl, mix the cornstarch, water, and soy sauce. Stir in the rice wine, sugar, and sesame oil, mixing well. Set aside.
2. In a large skillet or wok over medium-high heat, heat the canola oil.
3. Add the garlic, and cook until just fragrant, stirring constantly. Add the chicken, and cook for 1 minute, stirring, until the chicken is browned but not cooked through.
4. Add the cabbage, carrot, and scallions, and cook for 1 to 2 minutes, until the cabbage begins to wilt, and the chicken is cooked through.
5. Add the noodles and toss with the chicken and vegetables.
6. Pour in the sauce and stir to coat.
7. Add the bean sprouts and stir.
8. Remove from the heat and serve.

Nutrition:
Calories: 342, Fat: 18 g, Cholesterol: 31 mg, Carbs: 34 g, Fiber: 3 g, Protein: 13 g, Phosphorus: 169 mg, Potassium: 308 mg, Sodium: 289 mg

98.   Baked Herbed Chicken
Preparation Time: 10 minutes
Cooking Time: 40 minutes
Servings: 6
Ingredients:

- 4 tablespoons butter, at room temperature
- 4 garlic cloves, minced

- 1 tablespoon chopped fresh oregano
- 1 tablespoon chopped fresh parsley
- 1 teaspoon lemon zest
- 6 bone-in chicken thighs
- ¼ teaspoon freshly ground black pepper

Directions:

1. Preheat the oven to 425°F.
2. In a small bowl, add the butter, garlic, oregano, parsley, and lemon zest. Mix well.
3. Arrange the thighs on a baking tray, and gently peel back the skin, leaving it attached.
4. Brush the thigh meat with a couple of teaspoons of the butter mixture and replace the skin to cover the meat.
5. Season with pepper.
6. Bake for 40 minutes, until the skin, is crisp, and the juices run clear.
7. Let it rest for 5 minutes before serving.

Nutrition:
Calories: 226, Fat: 17 g, Cholesterol: 78 mg, Carbs: 1 g, Protein: 16 g, Phosphorus: 114 mg, Potassium: 158 mg, Sodium: 120 mg

99.   Chicken Satay with Peanut Sauce
Preparation Time: 10 minutes, plus 2 hours to marinate
Cooking Time: 10 minutes
Servings: 6
Ingredients:
For the Chicken:

- ½ cup plain, unsweetened yogurt
- 2 garlic cloves, minced
- 1-inch piece ginger, minced
- 2 teaspoons curry powder
- 1 pound boneless, skinless chicken breast, cut into strips
- 1 teaspoon canola oil

For the Peanut Sauce:

- ¾ cup smooth unsalted peanut butter
- 1 teaspoon soy sauce
- 1 tablespoon brown sugar
- Juice of 2 limes
- ½ teaspoon red chili flakes
- ¼ cup hot water
- Fresh cilantro leaves, chopped, for garnish
- Lime wedges, for garnish

Directions:
To Make the Chicken:

1. In a small bowl, add the yogurt, garlic, ginger, and curry powder. Stir to mix. Add the chicken strips to the marinade. Cover and refrigerate for 2 hours.
2. Thread the chicken pieces onto skewers.
3. Brush a grill pan with the oil, and heat on medium-high. Cook the chicken skewers on each side for 3 to 5 minutes, until cooked through.

To Make the Peanut Sauce:

1. In a food processor, combine the peanut butter, soy sauce, brown sugar, lime juice, red chili flakes, and hot water. Process until smooth. Transfer to a bowl, and sprinkle with the cilantro. Serve with the chicken satay along with lime wedges for squeezing over the skewers.

Nutrition:
Calories: 286, Fat: 18 g, Cholesterol: 43 mg, Carbs: 10 g, Fiber: 3 g, Protein: 25 g, Phosphorus: 33 mg, Potassium: 66 mg, Sodium: 201 mg

100. Chicken Breast and Bok Choy in Parchment
Preparation Time: 10 minutes
Cooking Time: 30 minutes
Servings: 4
Ingredients:

- 1 tablespoon Dijon mustard
- 1 tablespoon extra-virgin olive oil

- 1 tablespoon chopped fresh thyme leaves
- 2 cups thinly sliced bok choy
- 2 carrots, julienned
- 1 small leek, thinly sliced
- 4 boneless, skinless chicken breasts
- Freshly ground black pepper
- 4 lemon slices

Directions:

1. Preheat the oven to 425°F.
2. In a small bowl, mix the mustard, olive oil, and thyme.
3. Prepare four pieces of parchment paper by folding four 18-inch pieces in half and cutting them like you want to create a heart. Open each piece and lay flat.
4. In each piece of parchment, arrange ½ cup of bok choy, a small handful of carrots, and a few slices of leek. Place the chicken breast on top, and season with pepper.
5. Brush the marinade over the chicken breasts, and top each with a slice of lemon.
6. Fold the packets shut and fold the paper along the edges to the crease and seal the packages.
7. Cook for 20 minutes. Let rest for 5 minutes, and open carefully to serve.

Nutrition:
Calories: 164, Fat: 5 g, Cholesterol: 60 mg, Carbs: 8 g, Fiber: 2 g, Protein: 24 g, Phosphorus: 26 mg, Potassium: 187 mg, Sodium: 356 mg

101. One-Pan Curried Chicken Thighs and Cauliflower
Preparation Time: 10 minutes, plus 2 hours to marinate
Cooking Time: 40 minutes
Servings: 6
Ingredients:

- 3 tablespoons curry powder
- ½ teaspoon ground cumin
- ¼ teaspoon paprika
- ½ teaspoon freshly ground black pepper, divided
- 6 bone-in chicken thighs

- 4 teaspoons extra-virgin olive oil, divided
- 1 cauliflower head, cut into florets
- ½ teaspoon dried oregano
- Juice of 2 limes

Directions:

1. In a small bowl, mix the curry powder, cumin, paprika, and ¼ teaspoon of pepper.
2. In a medium bowl, drizzle 2 teaspoons of olive oil over the chicken thighs, and sprinkle with the curry mixture. Cover, refrigerate and marinate for at least 2 hours or up to overnight.
3. Preheat the oven to 400°F.
4. In a medium bowl, toss the cauliflower with the remaining 2 teaspoons of olive oil and the oregano. In a single layer, arrange the chicken and cauliflower on a baking sheet.
5. Bake for 40 minutes, stirring the cauliflower and flipping the chicken pieces once during cooking until the chicken is well browned, and its juices run clear.
6. Drizzle with the lime juice and serve.

Nutrition:

Calories: 175, Fat: 10 g, Cholesterol: 50 mg, Carbs: 8 g, Fiber: 3 g, Protein: 16 g, Phosphorus: 152 mg, Potassium: 486 mg, Sodium: 77 mg

Seafood Recipes

102. Fisherman's Stew
Preparation Time: 20 minutes
Cooking Time: 6-8 hours
Servings: 8
Ingredients:

- 1 fillet of seabass, cod, or other white fish, cubed
- 1 dozen each large shrimp, scallops, mussels & clams
- 1 28 ounces no-added salt crushed tomatoes with juice
- 1 8oz no-added salt tomato sauce
- ½ cup onion, chopped
- 1 cup dry white wine

- ⅓ cup olive oil
- 3 garlic cloves, minced
- ½ cup parsley, chopped
- 1 green pepper, chopped
- 1 hot pepper, chopped
- ½ tsp low sodium salt
- 1 tsp thyme
- 2 tsp basil
- 1 tsp oregano
- ½ tsp paprika
- ½ tsp cayenne pepper

Directions:

1. Place all ingredients except seafood in a 4 to 6-quart slow cooker and cover.
2. Cook on LOW for 6 to 8 hours.
3. Add the fish about 30 minutes towards the end of the cooking time and turn up the heat to HIGH.

Nutrition:
Calories: 434, Fat: 16 g, Carbs: 27 g, Protein: 39 g, Fiber: 4 g, Potassium: 714 mg, Sodium: 378 mg

103. Fish Chowder
Preparation Time: 15 minutes
Cooking Time: 6 hours
Servings: 6
Ingredients:

- 2lb white fish fillets, cut into 1-inch pieces
- ¼lb low-sodium bacon, diced
- 1 medium onion, chopped
- 4 medium red-skinned potatoes, peeled and cubed
- 2 cup water
- 1 low sodium salt
- ¼ tsp black pepper
- 1 12oz can evaporate milk

Directions:

1. Fry the bacon in a skillet for a few minutes with the onion.
2. Add the bacon to the slow cooker with the remaining ingredients except for the evaporated milk.
3. Cover and cook on HIGH for 5 to 6 hours.
4. Add the milk during the last hour of cooking.

Nutrition:
Calories: 311, Fat: 13 g, Carbs: 27 g, Protein: 14 g, Fiber: 12 g, Potassium: 911 mg, Sodium: 600 mg

104. Salmon with Caramelized Onions
Preparation Time: 20 minutes
Cooking Time: 6 hours
Servings: 6
Ingredients:

- 1lb salmon fillet, cut into small fillets
- 1 tbsp. extra-virgin olive oil
- ½ large onion, thinly sliced
- ¼ tsp ground ginger
- ¼ tsp dried dill
- ¼ tsp low-sodium salt
- ¼ tsp black pepper
- ½ lemon, thinly sliced

Directions:

1. Arrange the onions in the base of a 4 to 6-quart slow cooker.
2. Place each piece of salmon in an aluminum foil packet and sprinkle with spices and top with lemon slices.
3. Place the salmon packets on top of the onions in the slow cooker and cover.
4. Cook on LOW for 6 to 8 hours.
5. Serve the salmon on top of the onions.

Nutrition:
Calories: 215, Fat: 11 g, Carbs: 7 g, Protein: 24 g, Fiber: 2 g, Potassium: 520 mg, Sodium: 200 mg

105. Tuna and Red Pepper Stew
Preparation Time: 15 minutes

Cooking Time: 4 hours
Servings: 6
Ingredients:

- 1 tablespoon olive oil
- 1 onion, chopped
- 1 garlic clove, minced
- ¼ teaspoon red pepper flakes, or more to taste
- ½ cup dry white wine
- 1 (14-ounce) can diced tomatoes
- 1-pound baby red potatoes, scrubbed
- 1 teaspoon paprika
- 2 pounds' tuna fillet
- 2 roasted red bell peppers, seeded and cut into strips
- 3 tablespoons chopped cilantro for garnish

Directions:

1. Combine the oil, onions, garlic, red pepper flakes, wine, tomatoes, and potatoes, in a slow cooker. Cover and cook on HIGH for 2 hours. Add the tuna and the roasted peppers, season with the paprika, and replace the cover. Continue to cook on HIGH for another 2 hours or until the tuna is fully cooked.
2. Serve at once, topped with the cilantro.

Nutrition:
Calories: 107, Fat: 3 g, Cholesterol: 8 mg, Sodium: 200 mg, Carbs: 15 g, Fiber: 2 g, Protein: 5 g

106. Mediterranean Fish Stew
Preparation Time: 15 minutes
Cooking Time: 4 hours
Servings: 6
Ingredients:

- 1 onion, sliced
- 1 leek, white and light green portion, sliced thin
- 4 cloves garlic, minced
- ½ cup dry white wine

- ¼ cup water
- 4 bay leaves
- 1-piece orange peel, 2 inches, pith removed
- ½ teaspoon cracked black peppercorns
- 1 ½ pounds' haddock fillets
- 12 oz. shrimp (16/20), peeled and deveined
- 2 teaspoons extra-virgin olive oil for serving
- 2 tablespoons chopped parsley, flat-leaf

Directions:

1. Make a bed of the onion, leek, and garlic in the slow cooker. Add the wine and water to the cooker. Scatter the bay leaves, orange peel, and peppercorns on top. Cover the cooker and cook on HIGH for 2 hours. Add the fish and the shrimp, replace the cover, and cook on HIGH for an additional 2 hours or until the fish is cooked through and the shrimps are bright pink and opaque. Remove and discard the bay leaves and orange peel.
2. Serve the fish and shrimp in heated soup bowls topped with the cooking liquid and vegetables. Drizzle with olive oil and garnish with parsley.

Nutrition:
Calories: 207, Fat: 4 g, Cholesterol: 168 mg, Sodium: 536 mg, Carbs: 5 g, Fiber: 1 g, Protein: 32 g

107. Salmon Chowder with Sweet Potatoes and Corn
Preparation Time: 10 minutes
Cooking Time: 4 hours
Servings: 4
Ingredients:

- 1 tablespoon butter
- 1 onion, finely chopped
- 1 clove garlic, minced
- 2 teaspoons dill weed
- Freshly ground black pepper
- 3 tablespoons all-purpose flour
- 2 cups chicken broth (low sodium)

- 2 cups milk ()
- 2 cups diced sweet potatoes
- 1 ½ cups fresh or thawed frozen corn kernels
- 12 oz. salmon fillet, cut into chunks
- 1 teaspoon grated lemon zest
- 3 tablespoons lemon juice

Directions:

1. Melt the butter in a saucepan over medium heat. Add the onion, garlic, dill, and a pinch of pepper, sauté, stirring frequently until the onion is tender. Add the flour and stir until thick and pasty, about 2 minutes. Whisk in the broth until there are no lumps, then stir in the milk, and bring to a simmer. Pour into the slow cooker and add the sweet potatoes and corn. Cover with a lid and cook on LOW for 4 hours, until the potatoes are very tender.
2. Stir in the salmon, replace the lid, and cook on LOW for 20 minutes, or until the salmon is cooked (145°F) and very hot. Stir in the lemon zest and season to taste with lemon juice and additional pepper.
3. Serve in heated soup bowls.

Nutrition:
Calories: 391, Fat: 18 g, Cholesterol: 94 mg, Sodium: 320 mg, Carbs: 39 g, Fiber: 7 g, Protein: 37 g, Sugars: 17 g

108. Seafood Gumbo
Preparation Time: 25 minutes
Cooking Time: 5 hours
Servings: 6
Ingredients:

- 2 teaspoons olive oil
- ¼ cup minced turkey ham (low sodium)
- 2 stalks celery, sliced
- 1 medium onion, sliced
- 1 green bell pepper, chopped
- 2 cloves garlic, minced
- 2 cups chicken broth (low sodium)

- 1 (14-ounce) can diced tomatoes, including juices
- 1 teaspoon Worcestershire sauce
- ¼ teaspoon kosher salt
- 1 teaspoon dried thyme
- 1-pound shrimp (16/20), cleaned
- 1 pound fresh or frozen crabmeat, picked to remove cartilage
- 1 (10-ounce) package frozen okra, thawed

Directions:

1. Heat the oil in a sauté pan over medium-high heat. Add the ham and cook until crisp. With a slotted spoon, transfer the ham to a slow cooker.
2. Add the celery, onion, green pepper, and garlic to the sauté pan and cook over medium heat, stirring frequently, until the vegetables are tender about 10 minutes. Transfer to the cooker and add the broth, tomatoes and their juices, Worcestershire, salt, and thyme.
3. Cover and cook on LOW for 4 hours. Add the shrimp, crabmeat, and okra, and cook on HIGH for 20 minutes or until the shrimp is bright pink and firm.
4. Serve at once in heated soup bowls.

Nutrition:
Calories: 155, Fat: 5 g, Cholesterol: 207 mg, Sodium: 313 mg, Carbs: 16 g, Fiber: 5 g, Protein: 22 g, Sugars: 2 g

109. Peppered Balsamic Cod
Preparation Time: 10 minutes
Cooking Time: 2 hours
Servings: 4
Ingredients:

- 1 ½ pounds' cod filets
- 2 teaspoons olive oil
- 1 teaspoon lemon zest
- ½ teaspoon cracked black peppercorns
- 2 tablespoons balsamic vinegar, reduced to a syrup

Directions:

1. Cut a piece of foil large enough to wrap completely around the fish, or cut 4 smaller pieces to wrap the fish into individual packets. Brush the foil with 1 teaspoon of the oil. Arrange the fish in the center of the foil and brush with the remaining oil. Season evenly with the lemon zest and pepper. Drizzle with the balsamic vinegar. Fold the foil completely around the fish and crimp the edges to seal the package(s) completely.
2. Set the package in the slow cooker, cover with a lid, and cook on HIGH for 2 hours, or until the fish is completely cooked.
3. Serve at once.

Nutrition:
Calories: 201, Fat: 5 g, Cholesterol: 101 mg, Sodium: 121 mg, Carbs: 1 g, Fiber: 1 g, Protein: 39 g, Sugars: 1 g

110. Sesame Salmon Fillets
Preparation Time: 10 minutes
Cooking Time: 30 minutes
Servings: 4
Ingredients:

- 2 tbsp. Sesame Oil
- ¼ tsp. Sea Salt
- ¼ tsp. Black Pepper (cracked)
- 1 tbsp. Vinegar
- 4 tsp. Sesame Seeds (black)
- ¼ tsp. Ginger (ground)
- 4 skinless salmon fillets

Directions:

1. Coat the slow cooker with oil. Set the cooker on "high".
2. Place the salmon in the cooker. Drizzle the sesame seeds, pepper, salt, and ginger on the salmon.
3. Turn after 3 mins and repeat the procedure.
4. Add vinegar and cook on "high" for 20 mins.
5. Transfer the salmon to a plate. Serve immediately

Nutrition:

Calories: 319, Fats: 21 g, Cholesterol: 81 mg, Sodium: 204 mg, Carbs: 31 g, Fiber: 1 g, Protein: 31 g

111. Salmon and Sweet Potato Chowder
Preparation time: 15 minutes
Cooking Time: 4 hrs.
Servings: 4
Ingredients:

- 1 tbsp. Butter
- 1 minced clove of Garlic
- 1 chopped Onion
- 2 tsp. Dill Weed
- 3 tbsp. o all-purpose Flour
- Ground Black Pepper
- 2 cups Milk
- 2 cups Sweet Potatoes (diced)
- 2 cups Chicken Broth
- 1 ½ cups Corn Kernels
- 1 tsp. Lemon Zest
- 12 ounces sliced Salmon Fillets
- 3 tbsp. Lemon Juice

Directions:

1. Sauté pepper, dill, garlic, and onion in butter in a pan.
2. Add in the flour and cook for 2 mins.
3. Pour broth and then milk into the pan. Simmer.
4. Pour the mixture into the slow cooker and add the sweet potatoes.
5. Cook on "low" for 4 hrs.
6. Add in the salmon and cook again on "low" for 20 more mins.
7. Now, stir in the lemon zest, lemon juice, and pepper.
8. Serve hot in heated bowls.

Nutrition:
Calories: 391, Fat: 27 g, Cholesterol: 94 mg, Sodium: 320 mg, Carbs: 39 mg, Fiber: 7 g, Protein: 37 g

112. Curried Fish Cakes
Preparation Time: 10 minutes

Cooking Time: 18 minutes
Servings: 4
Ingredients:

- ¾ pound Atlantic cod, cubed
- 1 apple, peeled and cubed
- 1 tablespoon yellow curry paste
- 2 tablespoons cornstarch
- 1 tablespoon peeled grated ginger root
- 1 large egg
- 1 tablespoon freshly squeezed lemon juice
- ⅛ teaspoon freshly ground black pepper
- ½ cup crushed puffed rice cereal
- 1 tablespoon olive oil

Directions:

1. Put the cod, apple, curry, cornstarch, ginger, egg, lemon juice, and pepper in a blender or food processor and process until finely chopped. Avoid over-processing, or the mixture will become mushy.
2. Place the rice cereal on a shallow plate.
3. Form the mixture into 8 patties.
4. Dredge the patties in the rice cereal to coat.
5. Cook patties for 3 to 5 minutes per side, turning once until a meat thermometer registers 160°F.
6. Serve.

Nutrition:
Calories: 188, Fat: 6 g, Sodium: 150 mg, Potassium: 292 mg, Phosphorus: 150 mg, Carbs: 12 g, Fiber: 1 g, Protein: 21 g, Sugar: 5 g

113. Baked sole with caramelized onion
Preparation Time: 10 minutes
Cooking Time: 20 minutes
Servings: 4
Ingredients:

- 1 cup finely chopped onion
- ½ cup low-sodium vegetable broth

- 1 yellow summer squash, sliced
- 2 cups frozen broccoli florets
- 4 (3-ounce) fillets of sole
- Pinch salt
- 2 tablespoons olive oil
- Pinch baking soda
- 2 teaspoons avocado oil
- 1 teaspoon dried basil leaves

Directions:

1. Preheat the oven to 425°F.
2. Add the onions. Cook for 1 minute, then, stirring constantly, cook for another 4 minutes.
3. Remove the onions from the heat.
4. Pour the broth into a baking sheet with a lip and arrange the squash and broccoli on the sheet in a single layer. Top the vegetables with the fish. Sprinkle the fish with the salt and drizzle everything with olive oil.
5. Bake the fish and the vegetables for 10 minutes.
6. While the fish is baking, return the skillet with the onions to medium-high heat and stir in a pinch of baking soda.
7. Stir in the avocado oil and cook for 5 minutes, stirring frequently, until the onions are dark brown.
8. Transfer the onions to a plate.
9. Top the fish evenly with the onions. Sprinkle with the basil.
10. Return the fish to the oven and bake for 8-10 minutes.
11. Serve the fish on the vegetables.

Nutrition:
Calories: 202, Fat: 11 g, Sodium: 320 mg, Potassium: 537 mg, Phosphorus: 331 mg, Carbs: 10 g, Fiber: 3 g, Protein: 16 g, Sugar: 4 g

114. Thai tuna wraps
Preparation Time: 10 minutes
Cooking Time: 0 minutes
Servings: 4
Ingredients:

- ¼ cup unsalted peanut butter

- 2 tablespoons freshly squeezed lemon juice
- 1 teaspoon low-sodium soy sauce
- ½ teaspoon ground ginger
- ⅛ teaspoon cayenne pepper
- 1 (6-ounce) can no-salt-added or low-sodium chunk light tuna, drained
- 1 cup shredded red cabbage
- 2 scallions, white and green parts, chopped
- 1 cup grated carrots
- 8 butter lettuce leaves

Directions:

1. In a medium bowl, stir together the peanut butter, lemon juice, soy sauce, ginger, and cayenne pepper until well combined.
2. Stir in the tuna, cabbage, scallions, and carrots.
3. Divide the tuna filling evenly between the butter lettuce leaves and serve.

Nutrition:
Calories: 175, Fat: 10 g, Sodium: 98 mg, Potassium: 421 mg, Phosphorus: 153 mg, Carbs: 8 g, Fiber: 2 g, Protein: 17 g, Sugar: 4 g

115. Grilled fish and vegetable packets
Preparation Time: 15 minutes
Cooking Time: 12 minutes
Servings: 4
Ingredients:

- 1 (8-ounce) package sliced mushrooms
- 1 leek, white and green parts, chopped
- 1 cup frozen corn
- 4 (4-ounce) Atlantic cod fillets
- Juice of 1 lemon
- 3 tablespoons olive oil

Directions:

1. Prepare and preheat the grill to medium coals and set a grill 6 inches from the coals.

2. Tear off four 30-inch long strips of heavy-duty aluminum foil.
3. Arrange the mushrooms, leek, and corn in the center of each piece of foil and top with the fish.
4. Drizzle the packet contents evenly with the lemon juice and olive oil.
5. Bring the longer length sides of the foil together at the top and, holding the edges together, fold them over twice and then fold in the width sides to form a sealed packet with room for the steam.
6. Put the packets on the grill and grill for 10 to 12 minutes until the vegetables are tender-crisp and the fish flakes when tested with a fork. Be careful opening the packets because the escaping steam can be scalding.

Nutrition:
Calories: 267, Fat: 12 g, Sodium: 97 mg, Potassium: 582 mg, Phosphorus: 238 mg, Carbs: 13 g, Fiber: 2 g, Protein: 29 g, Sugar: 3 g

116.   **White fish soup**
Preparation Time: 15 minutes
Cooking Time: 20 minutes
Servings: 4
Ingredients:

- 2 tablespoons olive oil
- 1 onion, finely diced
- 1 green bell pepper, chopped
- 1 rib celery, thinly sliced
- 3 cups chicken broth, or more to taste
- ¼ cup chopped fresh parsley
- 1 ½ pounds' cod, cut into ¾-inch cubes
- Pepper to taste
- 1 dash red pepper flakes

Directions:

1. Heat oil in a soup pot over medium heat.
2. Add onion, bell pepper, and celery and cook until wilted, about 5 minutes.
3. Add broth and then bring to a simmer, about 5 minutes.

4. Cook 15 to 20 minutes.
5. Add cod, parsley, and red pepper flakes and simmer until fish flakes easily with a fork, 8 to 10 minutes more.
6. Season with black pepper.

Nutrition:

Calories: 117, Fat: 7.2 g, Cholesterol: 18 mg, Sodium: 37 mg, Carbs: 5.4 g, Fiber: 1.3 g, Sugars: 2.8 g, Protein: 8.1 g, Calcium: 23 mg, Iron: 1 mg, Potassium: 122 mg, Phosphorus: 111 mg

117. Lemon butter salmon
Preparation Time: 15 minutes
Cooking Time: 15 minutes
Servings: 6
Ingredients:

- 1 tablespoon butter
- 2 tablespoons olive oil
- 1 tablespoon Dijon mustard
- 1 tablespoon lemon juice
- 2 cloves garlic, crushed
- 1 teaspoon dried dill
- 1 teaspoon dried basil leaves
- 1 tablespoon capers
- 24-ounce salmon filet

Directions:

1. Put all the ingredients except the salmon in a saucepan over medium heat.
2. Bring to a boil and then simmer for 5 minutes.
3. Preheat your grill.
4. Create a packet using foil.
5. Place the sauce and salmon inside.
6. Seal the packet.
7. Grill for 12 minutes.

Nutrition:

Calories: 292, Protein: 22 g, Carbs: 2 g, Fat: 22 g, Cholesterol: 68 mg, Sodium: 190 mg, Potassium: 439 mg, Phosphorus: 280 mg, Calcium: 21 mg

118. Baked fish in cream sauce
Preparation Time: 10 minutes
Cooking Time: 40 minutes
Servings: 4
Ingredients:

- 1-pound haddock
- ½ cup all-purpose flour
- 2 tablespoons butter (unsalted)
- ¼ teaspoon pepper
- 2 cups fat-free nondairy creamer
- ¼ cup water

Directions:

1. Preheat your oven to 350 degrees f.
2. Spray baking pan with oil.
3. Sprinkle with a little flour.
4. Arrange fish on the pan
5. Season with pepper.
6. Sprinkle remaining flour on the fish.
7. Spread creamer on both sides of the fish.
8. Bake for 40 minutes or until golden.
9. Spread cream sauce on top of the fish before serving.

Nutrition:
Calories: 383, Protein: 24 g, Carbs: 46 g, Fat: 11 g, Cholesterol: 79 mg, Sodium: 253 mg, Potassium: 400 mg, Phosphorus: 266 mg, Calcium: 46 mg, Fiber: 0.4 g

119. Fish with mushrooms
Preparation Time: 5 minutes
Cooking Time: 16 minutes
Servings: 4
Ingredients:

- 1 pound cod fillet
- 2 tablespoons butter
- ¼ cup white onion, chopped
- 1 cup fresh mushrooms

- 1 teaspoon dried thyme

Directions:

1. Put the fish in a baking pan.
2. Preheat your oven to 450°F.
3. Melt the butter and cook onion and mushroom for 1 minute.
4. Spread mushroom mixture on top of the fish.
5. Season with thyme.
6. Bake in the oven for 15 minutes.

Nutrition:

Calories: 156, Protein: 21 g, Carbs: 3 g, Fat: 7 g, Cholesterol: 49 mg, Sodium: 110 mg, Potassium: 561 mg, Phosphorus: 225 mg, Calcium: 30 mg, Fiber: 0.5 g,

120. Salmon with spicy honey
Preparation Time: 15 minutes
Cooking Time: 8 minutes
Servings: 2
Ingredients:

- 16-ounce salmon fillet
- 3 tablespoon honey
- ¾ teaspoon lemon peel
- 3 bowls arugula salad
- ½ teaspoon black pepper
- ½ teaspoon garlic powder
- 2 teaspoons olive oil
- 1 teaspoon hot water

Directions:

1. Prepare a small bowl with some hot water and put in honey, grated lemon peel, ground pepper, and garlic powder.
2. Spread the mixture over salmon fillets.
3. Warm some olive oil at medium heat and add spiced salmon fillet and cook for 4 minutes.
4. Turn the fillets on one side than on the other side.

5. Continue to cook for the other 4 minutes at a reduced heat and try to check when the salmon fillets flake easily.

6. Put some arugula on each plate and add the salmon fillets on top, adding some aromatic herbs or some dill. Serve and enjoy!

Nutrition:
Calories: 320, Protein: 23 g, Sodium: 65 mg, Potassium: 450 mg, Phosphorus: 250 mg

121. Salmon with maple glaze
Preparation Time: 15 minutes
Cooking Time: 2 hours
Servings: 4
Ingredients:

- 1-pound salmon fillets
- 1 tablespoon green onion, chopped
- 1 tablespoon low sodium soy sauce
- 2 garlic cloves, pressed
- 2 tablespoons fresh cilantro
- 3 tablespoon lemon juice (or juice of 1 lemon)
- 3 tablespoon maple syrup

Directions:

1. Combine all ingredients except for salmon.
2. Put salmon on a platter and then pour marinade over fillets. Let it marinate for 2 hours or more.
3. Preheat broiler.
4. Remove salmon from marinade.
5. Place salmon on the bottom rack and broil for 10 minutes. Do not turn over.
6. Serve hot/cold with a wedge of lemon.

Nutrition:
Calories: 220, Carbs: 12 g, Protein: 24 g, Fats: 8 g, Phosphorus: 374 mg, Potassium: 440 mg, Sodium: 621 mg

122. Shrimp Paella
Preparation Time: 5 minutes
Cooking Time: 10 minutes

Servings: 2
Ingredients:

- 1 cup cooked brown rice
- 1 chopped red onion
- 1 teaspoon paprika
- 1 chopped garlic clove
- 1 tablespoon olive oil
- 6 oz. frozen cooked shrimp
- 1 deseeded and sliced chili pepper
- 1 tablespoon oregano

Directions:

1. Heat the olive oil in a large pan on medium-high heat.
2. Add the onion and garlic and sauté for 2-3 minutes until soft.
3. Now add the shrimp and sauté for a further 5 minutes or until hot through.
4. Now add the herbs, spices, chili, and rice with ½ cup boiling water.
5. Stir until everything is warm and the water has been absorbed.
6. Plate up and serve.

Nutrition:
Calories: 221, Protein: 17 g, Carbs: 31 g, Fat: 8 g, Sodium: 235 mg, Potassium: 176 mg, Phosphorus: 189 mg

123. Salmon and Pesto Salad
Preparation Time: 5 minutes
Cooking Time: 15 minutes
Servings: 2
Ingredients:
For the pesto:

- 1 minced garlic clove
- ½ cup fresh arugula
- ¼ cup extra virgin olive oil
- ½ cup fresh basil
- 1 teaspoon black pepper

For the salmon:

- 4 oz. skinless salmon fillet
- 1 tablespoon coconut oil
- For the salad:
- ½ juiced lemon
- 2 sliced radishes
- ½ cup iceberg lettuce
- 1 teaspoon black pepper

Directions:

1. Prepare the pesto by blending all the ingredients for the pesto in a food processor or by grinding with a pestle and mortar. Set aside.
2. Add a skillet to the stove on medium-high heat and melt the coconut oil.
3. Add the salmon to the pan.
4. Cook for 7-8 minutes and turn over.
5. Cook for a further 3-4 minutes or until cooked through.
6. Remove fillets from the skillet and allow to rest.
7. Mix the lettuce and the radishes and squeeze over the juice of ½ lemon.
8. Flake the salmon with a fork and mix through the salad.
9. Toss to coat and sprinkle with a little black pepper to serve.

Nutrition:
Calories: 221, Protein: 13 g, Carbs: 1 g, Fat: 34 g, Sodium: 80 mg, Potassium: 119 mg, Phosphorus: 158 mg

124. Baked Fennel and Garlic Sea Bass
Preparation Time: 5 minutes
Cooking Time: 15 minutes
Servings: 2
Ingredients:

- 1 lemon
- ½ sliced fennel bulb
- 6 oz. sea bass fillets
- 1 teaspoon black pepper

- 2 garlic cloves

Directions:

1. Preheat the oven to 375°F/Gas Mark 5.
2. Sprinkle black pepper over the Sea Bass.
3. Slice the fennel bulb and garlic cloves.
4. Add 1 salmon fillet and half the fennel and garlic to one sheet of baking paper or tin foil.
5. Squeeze in ½ lemon juices.
6. Repeat for the other fillet.
7. Fold and add to the oven for 12-15 minutes or until fish is thoroughly cooked through.
8. Meanwhile, add boiling water to your couscous, cover, and allow to steam.
9. Serve with your choice of rice or salad.

Nutrition:
Calories: 221, Protein: 14 g, Carbs: 3 g, Fat: 2 g, Sodium: 119 mg, Potassium: 398 mg, Phosphorus: 149 mg

125. Lemon, Garlic & Cilantro Tuna and Rice
Preparation Time: 5 minutes
Cooking Time: 0 minutes
Servings: 2
Ingredients:

- ½ cup arugula
- 1 tablespoon extra-virgin olive oil
- 1 cup cooked rice
- 1 teaspoon black pepper
- ¼ finely diced red onion
- 1 juiced lemon
- 3 oz. canned tuna
- 2 tablespoons chopped fresh cilantro

Directions:

1. Mix the olive oil, pepper, cilantro, and red onion in a bowl.

2. Stir in the tuna, cover, and leave in the fridge for as long as possible (if you can) or serve immediately.

3. When ready to eat, serve up with the cooked rice and arugula!

Nutrition:

Calories: 221, Protein: 11 g, Carbs: 26 g, Fat: 7 g, Sodium: 143 mg, Potassium: 197 mg, Phosphorus: 182 mg

126. Cod & Green Bean Risotto
Preparation Time: 4 minutes
Cooking Time: 40 minutes
Servings: 2
Ingredients:

- ½ cup arugula
- 1 finely diced white onion
- 4 oz. cod fillet
- 1 cup white rice
- 2 lemon wedges
- 1 cup boiling water
- ¼ teaspoon black pepper
- 1 cup low sodium chicken broth
- 1 tablespoon extra-virgin olive oil
- ½ cup green beans

Directions:

1. Heat the oil in a large pan on medium heat.
2. Sauté the chopped onion for 5 minutes until soft before adding in the rice and stirring for 1-2 minutes.
3. Combine the broth with boiling water.
4. Add half of the liquid to the pan and stir slowly.
5. Slowly add the rest of the liquid whilst continuously stirring for up to 20-30 minutes.
6. Stir in the green beans to the risotto.
7. Place the fish on top of the rice, cover, and steam for 10 minutes.
8. Ensure the water does not dry out and keep topping up until the rice is cooked thoroughly.
9. Use your fork to break up the fish fillets and stir into the rice.

10. Sprinkle with freshly ground pepper and a squeeze of fresh lemon to serve.
11. Garnish with the lemon wedges and serve with the arugula.

Nutrition:
Calories: 221, Protein: 12 g, Carbs: 29 g, Fat: 8 g, Sodium: 398 mg, Potassium: 347 mg, Phosphorus: 241 mg

127. Mixed Pepper Stuffed River Trout
Preparation Time: 5 minutes
Cooking Time: 20 minutes
Servings: 4
Ingredients:

- 1 whole river trout
- 1 teaspoon thyme
- ¼ diced yellow pepper
- 1 cup baby spinach leaves
- ¼ diced green pepper
- 1 juiced lime
- ¼ diced red pepper
- 1 teaspoon oregano
- 1 teaspoon extra virgin olive oil
- 1 teaspoon black pepper

Directions:

1. Preheat the broiler /grill on high heat.
2. Lightly oil a baking tray.
3. Mix all the ingredients apart from the trout and lime.
4. Slice the trout lengthways (there should be an opening here from where it was gutted) and stuff the mixed ingredients inside.
5. Squeeze the lime juice over the fish and then place the lime wedges on the tray.
6. Place under the broiler on the baking tray and broil for 15-20 minutes or until fish is thoroughly cooked through and flakes easily.
7. Enjoy the dish as it is, or with a side helping of rice or salad.

Nutrition:
Calories: 290, Protein: 15 g, Fat: 7 g, Sodium: 43 mg, Potassium: 315 mg, Phosphorus: 189 mg

128. Haddock & Buttered Leeks
Preparation Time: 5 minutes
Cooking Time: 15 minutes
Servings: 2
Ingredients:

- 1 tablespoon unsalted butter
- 1 sliced leek
- ¼ teaspoon black pepper
- 2 teaspoons chopped parsley
- 6 oz. haddock fillets
- ½ juiced lemon

Directions:

1. Preheat the oven to 375°F/Gas Mark 5.
2. Add the haddock fillets to baking or parchment paper and sprinkle with the black pepper.
3. Squeeze over the lemon juice and wrap into a parcel.
4. Bake the parcel on a baking tray for 10-15 minutes or until the fish is thoroughly cooked through.
5. Meanwhile, heat the butter over medium-low heat in a small pan.
6. Add the leeks and parsley and sauté for 5-7 minutes until soft.
7. Serve the haddock fillets on a bed of buttered leeks and enjoy!

Nutrition:
Calories: 124, Protein: 15 g, Fat: 7 g, Sodium: 161 mg, Potassium: 251 mg, Phosphorus: 220 mg

129. Thai Spiced Halibut
Preparation Time: 5 minutes
Cooking Time: 20 minutes
Servings: 2
Ingredients:

- 2 tablespoons coconut oil

- 1 cup white rice
- ¼ teaspoon black pepper
- ½ diced red chili
- 1 tablespoon fresh basil
- 2 pressed garlic cloves
- 4 oz. halibut fillet
- 1 halved lime
- 2 sliced green onions
- 1 lime leaf

Directions:

1. Preheat oven to 400°F/Gas Mark 5.
2. Add half of the ingredients into baking paper and fold into a parcel.
3. Repeat for your second parcel.
4. Add to the oven for 15-20 minutes or until fish is thoroughly cooked through.
5. Serve with cooked rice.

Nutrition:
Calories: 311, Protein: 16 g, Carbs: 17 g, Fat: 15 g, Sodium: 31 mg, Potassium: 418 mg, Phosphorus: 257 mg

130. Homemade Tuna Niçoise
Preparation Time: 5 minutes
Cooking Time: 10 minutes
Servings: 2
Ingredients:

- 1 egg
- ½ cup green beans
- ¼ sliced cucumber
- 1 juiced lemon
- 1 teaspoon black pepper
- ¼ sliced red onion
- 1 tablespoon olive oil
- 1 tablespoon capers
- 4 oz. drained canned tuna
- 4 iceberg lettuce leaves

- 1 teaspoon chopped fresh cilantro

Directions:

1. Prepare the salad by washing and slicing the lettuce, cucumber, and onion.
2. Add to a salad bowl.
3. Mix 1 tablespoon oil with the lemon juice, cilantro, and capers for a salad dressing. Set aside.
4. Boil a pan of water on high heat then lower to simmer and add the egg for 6 minutes. (Steam the green beans over the same pan in a steamer/colander for 6 minutes).
5. Remove the egg and rinse under cold water.
6. Peel before slicing in half.
7. Mix the tuna, salad, and dressing together in a salad bowl.
8. Toss to coat.
9. Top with the egg and serve with a sprinkle of black pepper.

Nutrition:
Calories: 199, Protein: 19 g, Carbs: 7 g, Fat: 8 g, Sodium: 466 mg, Potassium: 251 mg, Phosphorus: 211 mg

131. Monk-Fish Curry
Preparation Time: 5 minutes
Cooking Time: 20 minutes
Servings: 2
Ingredients:

- 1 garlic clove
- 3 finely chopped green onions
- 1 teaspoon grated ginger
- 1 cup water.
- 2 teaspoons chopped fresh basil
- 1 cup cooked rice noodles
- 1 tablespoon coconut oil
- ½ sliced red chili
- 4 oz. Monkfish fillet
- ½ finely sliced stick lemongrass
- 2 tablespoons chopped shallots

Directions:

1. Slice the Monkfish into bite-size pieces.
2. Using a pestle and mortar or food processor, crush the basil, garlic, ginger, chili, and lemongrass to form a paste.
3. Heat the oil in a large wok or pan over medium-high heat and add the shallots.
4. Now add the water to the pan and bring to a boil.
5. Add the Monkfish, lower the heat, and cover to simmer for 10 minutes or until cooked through.
6. Enjoy with rice noodles and scatter with green onions to serve.

Nutrition:
Calories: 249, Protein: 12 g, Carbs: 30 g, Fat: 10 g, Sodium: 32 mg, Potassium: 398 mg, Phosphorus: 190 mg

132. Grilled Shrimp with Cucumber Lime Salsa
Preparation Time: 15 minutes
Cooking Time: 10 minutes
Servings: 4
Ingredients:

- 2 tbsp. Olive oil
- 6 ounces large shrimp, peeled and deveined, tails left on
- 1 tsp. Minced Garlic
- ½ cup Chopped English cucumber
- ½ cup Chopped mango
- Zest of 1 lime
- Juice of 1 lime
- Ground black pepper
- Lime wedges for garnish

Directions:

1. Soak 4 wooden skewers in water for 30 minutes.
2. Preheat the barbecue to medium heat.
3. In a bowl, toss together the olive oil, shrimp, and garlic.
4. Thread the shrimp onto the skewers, about 4 shrimp per skewer.

5. In a bowl, stir together the mango, cucumber, lime zest, and lime juice, and season the salsa lightly with pepper. Set aside.
6. Grill the shrimp for 10 minutes, turning once or until the shrimp is opaque and cooked through.
7. Season the shrimp lightly with pepper.
8. Serve the shrimp on the cucumber salsa with lime wedges on the side.

Nutrition:
Calories: 120, Fat: 8 g, Sodium: 60 mg, Carbs: 4 g, Protein: 9 g

Vegetarian & Vegan Recipes

133. Cauliflower Rice
Preparation Time: 10 minutes
Cooking Time: 10 minutes
Servings: 4
Ingredients:

- 1 head cauliflower, sliced into florets
- 1 tablespoon butter
- Black pepper to taste
- ¼ teaspoon garlic powder
- ¼ teaspoon herb seasoning blend

Directions:

1. Put cauliflower florets in a food processor.
2. Pulse until consistency is like grain.
3. In a pan over medium heat, melt the butter and add the spices.
4. Toss cauliflower rice and cook for 10 minutes.
5. Fluff using a fork before serving.

Nutrition:
Calories: 47, Protein: 1 g, Carbs: 4 g, Fat: 3 g, Cholesterol: 8 mg, Sodium: 43 mg, Potassium: 206 mg, Phosphorus: 31 mg, Calcium: 16 mg, Fiber: 1.4 g

134. Eggplant Fries
Preparation Time: 10 minutes

Cooking Time: 5 minutes
Servings: 6
Ingredients:

- 2 eggs, beaten
- 1 cup almond milk
- 1 teaspoon hot sauce
- ¾ cup cornstarch
- 3 teaspoons dry ranch seasoning mix
- ¾ cup dry breadcrumbs
- 1 eggplant, sliced into strips
- ½ cup oil

Directions:

1. In a bowl, mix eggs, milk and hot sauce.
2. In a dish, mix cornstarch, seasoning, and breadcrumbs.
3. Dip first the eggplant strips in the egg mixture.
4. Coat each strip with the cornstarch mixture.
5. Pour oil into a pan over medium heat.
6. Once hot, add the fries and cook for 3 minutes or until golden.

Nutrition:
Calories: 234, Protein: 7 g, Carbs: 25 g, Fat: 13 g, Cholesterol: 48 mg, Sodium: 212 mg, Potassium: 215 mg, Phosphorus: 86 mg, Calcium: 70 mg, Fiber: 2.1 g

135. Seasoned Green Beans
Preparation Time: 10 minutes
Cooking Time: 10 minutes
Servings: 4
Ingredients:

- 10-ounce green beans
- 4 teaspoons butter
- ¼ cup onion, chopped
- ½ cup red bell pepper, chopped
- 1 teaspoon dried dill weed
- 1 teaspoon dried parsley
- ¼ teaspoon black pepper

Directions:

1. Boil green beans in a pot of water. Drain.
2. In a pan over medium heat, melt the butter and cook onion and bell pepper.
3. Season with dill and parsley.
4. Put the green beans back to the skillet.
5. Sprinkle pepper on top before serving.

Nutrition:
Calories: 67, Protein: 2 g, Carbs: 8 g, Fat: 3 g, Sodium: 55 mg, Potassium: 194 mg, Phosphorus: 32 mg, Calcium: 68 mg, Fiber: 4.0 g

136. Grilled Squash
Preparation Time: 10 minutes
Cooking Time: 6 minutes
Servings: 8
Ingredients:

- 4 zucchinis, rinsed, drained, and sliced
- 4 crookneck squash, rinsed, drained, and sliced
- Cooking spray
- ¼ teaspoon garlic powder
- ¼ teaspoon black pepper

Directions:

1. Arrange squash on a baking sheet.
2. Spray with oil.
3. Season with garlic powder and pepper.
4. Grill for 3 minutes per side or until tender but not too soft.

Nutrition:
Calories: 17, Protein: 1 g, Carbs: 3 g, Sodium: 6 mg, Potassium: 262 mg, Phosphorus: 39 mg, Calcium: 16 mg, Fiber: 1.1 g

137. Delicious Vegetarian Lasagna
Preparation Time: 10 minutes
Cooking Time: 1 hour
Servings: 4
Ingredients:

- 1 teaspoon basil
- 1 tablespoon olive oil
- ½ sliced red pepper
- 3 lasagna sheets
- ½ diced red onion
- ¼ teaspoon black pepper
- 1 cup rice milk
- 1 minced garlic clove
- 1 cup sliced eggplant
- ½ sliced zucchini
- ½ pack soft tofu
- 1 teaspoon oregano

Directions:

1. Preheat oven to 325°F/Gas Mark 3.
2. Slice zucchini, eggplant, and pepper into vertical strips.
3. Add the rice milk and tofu to a food processor and blitz until smooth. Set aside.
4. Heat the oil in a skillet over medium heat and add the onions and garlic for 3-4 minutes or until soft.
5. Sprinkle in the herbs and pepper and allow to stir through for 5-6 minutes until hot.
6. Into a lasagna or suitable oven dish, layer 1 lasagna sheet, then ⅓ the eggplant, followed by ⅓ zucchini, then ⅓ pepper before pouring over ⅓ of tofu white sauce.
7. Repeat for the next 2 layers, finishing with the white sauce.
8. Add to the oven for 40-50 minutes or until veg is soft and can easily be sliced into Servings.

Nutrition:
Calories: 235, Protein: 5 g, Carbs: 10g, Fat: 9 g, Sodium: 35 mg, Potassium: 129 mg, Phosphorus: 66 mg
138. Chili Tofu Noodles
Preparation Time: 5 minutes
Cooking Time: 15 minutes
Servings: 4
Ingredients:

- ½ diced red chili
- 2 cups of rice noodles
- ½ juiced lime
- 6 ounce pressed and cubed silken firm tofu
- 1 teaspoon grated fresh ginger
- 1 tablespoon coconut oil
- 1 cup green beans
- 1 minced garlic clove

Directions:

1. Steam the green beans for 10-12 minutes or according to package directions and drain.
2. Cook the noodles in a pot of boiling water for 10-15 minutes or according to package directions.
3. Meanwhile, heat a wok or skillet on high heat and add coconut oil.
4. Now add the tofu, chili flakes, garlic, and ginger, and sauté for 5-10 minutes.
5. After doing that, drain in the noodles along with the green beans and lime juice then add it to the wok.
6. Toss to coat.
7. Serve hot!

Nutrition:
Calories: 246, Protein: 10 g, Carbs: 28g, Fat: 12 g, Sodium: 25 mg, Potassium: 126 mg, Phosphorus: 79 mg

139. Curried Cauliflower
Preparation Time: 5 minutes
Cooking Time: 20 minutes
Servings: 4
Ingredients:

- 1 teaspoon turmeric
- 1 diced onion
- 1 tablespoon chopped fresh cilantro
- 1 teaspoon cumin
- ½ diced chili
- ½ cup water

- 1 minced garlic clove
- 1 tablespoon coconut oil
- 1 teaspoon garam masala
- 2 cups cauliflower florets

Directions:

1. Add the oil to a skillet on medium heat.
2. Sauté the onion and garlic for 5 minutes until soft.
3. Add in the cumin, turmeric, and garam masala and stir to release the aromas.
4. Now add the chili to the pan along with the cauliflower.
5. Stir to coat.
6. Pour in the water and reduce the heat to a simmer for 15 minutes.
7. Garnish with cilantro to serve.

Nutrition:
Calories: 108, Protein: 2 g, Carbs: 11 g, Fat: 7 g, Sodium: 35 mg, Potassium: 328 mg, Phosphorus: 39 mg

140. Elegant Veggie Tortillas
Preparation Time: 30 minutes
Cooking Time: 15 minutes
Servings: 12
Ingredients:

- 1½ cups of chopped broccoli florets
- 1½ cups of chopped cauliflower florets
- 1 tablespoon of water
- 2 teaspoon of canola oil
- 1½ cups of chopped onion
- 1 minced garlic clove
- 2 tablespoons of finely chopped fresh parsley
- 1 cup of low-cholesterol liquid egg substitute
- Freshly ground black pepper, to taste
- 4 (6-ounce) warmed corn tortillas

Directions:

1. In a microwave bowl, place broccoli, cauliflower, and water, and microwave, covered for about 3-5 minutes.
2. Remove from microwave and drain any liquid.
3. Heat oil on medium heat.
4. Add onion and sauté for about 4-5 minutes.
5. Add garlic and then sauté it for about 1 minute.
6. Stir in broccoli, cauliflower, parsley, egg substitute, and black pepper.
7. Reduce the heat and it to simmer for about 10 minutes.
8. Remove from heat and keep aside to cool slightly.
9. Place broccoli mixture over ¼ of each tortilla.
10. Fold the outside edges inward and roll up like a burrito.
11. Secure each tortilla with toothpicks to secure the filling.
12. Cut each tortilla in half and serve.

Nutrition:
Calories: 217, Fat: 3.3 g, Carbs: 41 g, Protein: 8.1 g, Fiber: 6.3 g, Potassium: 289 mg, Sodium: 87 mg

141. Simple Broccoli Stir-Fry
Preparation Time: 40 minutes
Cooking Time: 15 minutes
Servings: 4
Ingredients:

- 1 tablespoon of olive oil
- 1 minced garlic clove
- 2 cups of broccoli florets
- 2 tablespoons of water

Directions:

1. Heat oil on medium heat.
2. Add garlic and then sauté for about 1 minute.
3. Add the broccoli and stir fry for about 2 minutes.
4. Stir in water and stir fry for about 4-5 minutes.
5. Serve warm.

Nutrition:
Calories: 47, Fat: 3.6 g, Carbs: 3.3 g, Protein: 1.3 g, Fiber: 1.2 g, Potas-

sium: 147 mg, Sodium: 15 mg

142. Braised Cabbage
Preparation Time: 30 minutes
Cooking Time: 15 minutes
Servings: 4
Ingredients:

- 1½ teaspoon of olive oil
- 2 minced garlic cloves
- 1 thinly sliced onion
- 3 cups of chopped green cabbage
- 1 cup of low-sodium vegetable broth
- Freshly ground black pepper, to taste

Directions:

1. In a large skillet, heat oil on medium-high heat.
2. Add garlic and then sauté for about 1 minute.
3. Add onion and sauté for about 4-5 minutes.
4. Add cabbage and sauté for about 3-4 minutes.
5. Stir in broth and black pepper and immediately, reduce the heat to low.
6. Cook, covered for about 20 minutes.
7. Serve warm.

Nutrition:
Calories: 45, Fat: 1.8 g, Carbs: 6.6 g, Protein: 1.1 g, Fiber: 1.9 g, Potassium: 136 mg, Sodium: 46 mg

143. Mashed Cauliflower
Preparation Time: 10 minutes
Cooking Time: 10 minutes
Servings: 3
Ingredients:

- 1 cauliflower head
- 1 tablespoon olive oil
- ½ tsp salt
- ¼ tsp dill
- Pepper to taste

- 2 tbsp. low-fat milk

Directions:

1. Bring a small pot of water to a boil.
2. Chop cauliflower in florets.
3. Add florets to boiling water and boil uncovered for 5 minutes. Turn off the fire and let it sit for 5 minutes more.
4. In a blender, add all ingredients except for cauliflower and blend to mix well.
5. Drain cauliflower well and add it into the blender. Puree until smooth and creamy.
6. Serve and enjoy.

Nutrition:
Calories: 78, Fat: 5 g, Carbs: 6 g, Protein: 2 g, Sugar: 3 g, Fiber: 2 g, Sodium: 420 mg, Potassium: 327 mg

144. Stir-Fried Eggplant
Preparation Time: 10 minutes
Cooking Time: 10 minutes
Servings: 2
Ingredients:

- 1 tablespoon coconut oil
- 2 eggplants, sliced into 3-inch in length
- 4 cloves of garlic, minced
- 1 onion, chopped
- 1 teaspoon ginger, grated
- 1 teaspoon lemon juice, freshly squeezed
- ½ tsp salt
- ½ tsp pepper

Directions:

1. Heat oil in a nonstick saucepan.
2. Pan-fry the eggplants for 2 minutes on all sides.
3. Add the garlic and onions until fragrant, around 3 minutes.
4. Stir in the ginger, salt, pepper, and lemon juice.

5. Add a ½ cup of water and bring to a simmer. Cook until eggplant is tender.

Nutrition:
Calories: 232, Fat: 8 g, Carbs: 41 g, Protein: 7 g, Sugar: 22 g, Fiber: 18 g, Sodium: 596 mg, Potassium: 1404 mg

145. Sautéed Garlic Mushrooms
Preparation Time: 10 minutes
Cooking Time: 10 minutes
Servings: 4
Ingredients:

- 1 tablespoon olive oil
- 3 cloves of garlic, minced
- 16 oz. fresh brown mushrooms, sliced
- 7 oz. fresh shiitake mushrooms, sliced
- ½ tsp salt
- ½ tsp pepper or more to taste

Directions:

1. Place a nonstick saucepan on medium-high fire and heat pan for 1 minute.
2. Add oil and heat for 2 minutes.
3. Stir in garlic and sauté for 1 minute.
4. Add remaining ingredients and stir fry until soft and tender, around 5 minutes.
5. Turn off the fire, let mushrooms rest while the pan is covered for 5 minutes.
6. Serve and enjoy.

Nutrition:
Calories: 95, Fat: 4 g, Carbs: 14 g, Protein: 3 g, Sugar: 5 g, Fiber: 4 g, Sodium: 296 mg, Potassium: 490 mg

146. Stir-Fried Asparagus and Bell Pepper
Preparation Time: 10 minutes
Cooking Time: 10 minutes
Servings: 6
Ingredients:

- 1 tablespoon olive oil
- 4 cloves of garlic, minced
- 1-pound fresh asparagus spears, trimmed
- 2 large red bell peppers, seeded and julienned
- ½ teaspoon thyme
- 5 tablespoons water
- ½ tsp salt
- ½ tsp pepper or more to taste

Directions:

1. Place a nonstick saucepan on high fire and heat pan for 1 minute.
2. Add oil and heat for 2 minutes.
3. Stir in garlic and sauté for 1 minute.
4. Add remaining ingredients and stir fry until soft and tender, around 6 minutes.
5. Turn off the fire, let veggies rest while the pan is covered for 5 minutes.
6. Serve and enjoy.

Nutrition:

Calories: 45, Fat: 2 g, Carbs: 5 g, Protein: 2 g, Sugar: 2 g, Fiber: 2 g, Sodium: 482 mg, Potassium: 219 mg

147. Stir-fried Brussels Sprouts and Pecans
Preparation Time: 10 minutes
Cooking Time: 10 minutes
Servings: 7
Ingredients:

- 1 ½ pound fresh Brussels sprouts, trimmed and halved
- 1 tablespoon olive oil
- 4 cloves of garlic, minced
- 3 tablespoons water
- ¼ tsp salt
- ½ tsp pepper or more to taste
- ½ cup chopped pecans

Directions:

1. Place a nonstick saucepan on high fire and heat pan for 1 minute.
2. Add oil and heat for 2 minutes.
3. Stir in garlic and sauté for 1 minute.
4. Add remaining ingredients and stir fry until soft and tender, around 6 minutes.
5. Turn off the fire, let veggies rest while the pan is covered for 5 minutes.
6. Serve and enjoy.

Nutrition:

Calories: 112, Fat: 7 g, Carbs: 11 g, Protein: 4 g, Sugar: 4 g, Fiber: 3 g, Sodium: 108 mg, Potassium: 425 mg

148. Stir-Fried Kale
Preparation Time: 10 minutes
Cooking Time: 10 minutes
Servings: 6
Ingredients:

- 1 tablespoon coconut oil
- 2 cloves of garlic, minced
- 1 onion, chopped
- 2 teaspoons crushed red pepper flakes
- 4 cups kale, chopped
- 2 tbsp. water
- Salt and pepper to taste

Directions:

1. Place a nonstick saucepan on high fire and heat pan for 1 minute.
2. Add oil and heat for 2 minutes.
3. Stir in garlic and sauté for 1 minute. Add onions and stir fry for another minute.
4. Add remaining ingredients and stir fry until soft and tender, around 4 minutes.
5. Turn off the fire, let veggies rest while the pan is covered for 3 minutes.
6. Serve and enjoy.

Nutrition:
Calories: 37, Fat: 2 g, Carbs: 4 g, Protein: 1 g, Sugar: 1 g, Fiber: 1 g, Sodium: 6 mg, Potassium: 111 mg

149. Stir-Fried Bok Choy
Preparation Time: 10 minutes
Cooking Time: 12 minutes
Servings: 1
Ingredients:

- 1 tablespoon coconut oil
- 4 cloves of garlic, minced
- 1 onion, chopped
- 2 heads bok choy, rinsed and chopped
- ¼ tsp salt
- ½ tsp pepper or more to taste
- 1 tablespoon sesame seeds

Directions:

1. Place a nonstick saucepan on high fire and heat pan for 1 minute.
2. Add sesame seeds and toast for 1 minute. Transfer to a bowl.
3. In the same pan, add oil and heat for 2 minutes.
4. Stir in garlic and sauté for 1 minute. Add onions and stir fry for another minute.
5. Add remaining ingredients and stir fry until soft and tender, around 4 minutes.
6. Turn off the fire, let veggies rest while the pan is covered for 3 minutes.
7. Serve and enjoy.

Nutrition:
Calories: 334, Fat: 20 g, Carbs: 36 g, Protein: 12 g, Sugar: 6 g, Fiber: 14 g, Sodium: 731 mg, Potassium: 1043 mg

150. Vegetable Curry
Preparation Time: 10 minutes
Cooking Time: 20 minutes
Servings: 4
Ingredients:

- 1 tablespoon coconut oil
- 1 medium onion, chopped
- 1 teaspoon minced garlic
- 1 teaspoon minced ginger
- 2 cup broccoli florets
- 2 cups fresh spinach leaves
- 1 tablespoon garam masala
- ½ cup coconut milk
- ½ tsp salt
- ½ tsp pepper

Directions:

1. Place a nonstick pot on high fire and heat pot for 1 minute.
2. Add oil and heat for 2 minutes.
3. Stir in garlic and ginger, sauté for 1 minute. Add onions and garam masala and stir fry for another minute.
4. Add remaining ingredients, except for spinach leaves, and simmer for 10 minutes.
5. Stir in spinach leaves, turn off the fire, let veggies rest while the pot is covered for 5 minutes.
6. Serve and enjoy.

Nutrition:
Calories: 121, Fat: 11 g, Carbs: 6 g, Protein: 2 g, Sugar: 3 g, Fiber: 2 g, Sodium: 315 mg, Potassium: 266 mg

151. Braised Carrots 'n Kale
Preparation Time: 10 minutes
Cooking Time: 10 minutes
Servings: 2
Ingredients:

- 1 tablespoon coconut oil
- 1 onion, sliced thinly
- 5 cloves of garlic, minced
- 3 medium carrots, sliced thinly
- 10 ounces of kale, chopped
- ½ cup water
- Salt and pepper to taste

- A dash of red pepper flakes

Directions:

1. Heat oil in a skillet over medium flame and sauté the onion and garlic until fragrant.
2. Toss in the carrots and stir for 1 minute. Add the kale and water. Season with salt and pepper to taste.
3. Close the lid and allow to simmer for 5 minutes.
4. Sprinkle with red pepper flakes.
5. Serve and enjoy.

Nutrition:
Calories: 161, Fat: 8 g, Carbs: 20 g, Protein: 8 g, Sugar: 6 g, Fiber: 6 g, Sodium: 63 mg, Potassium: 900 mg

152. Butternut Squash Hummus
Preparation Time: 10 minutes
Cooking Time: 15 minutes
Servings: 8
Ingredients:

- 2 pounds butternut squash, seeded and peeled
- 1 tablespoon olive oil
- ¼ cup tahini
- 2 tablespoons lemon juice
- 2 cloves of garlic, minced
- Salt and pepper to taste

Directions:

1. Heat the oven to 300°F.
2. Coat the butternut squash with olive oil.
3. Place in a baking dish and bake for 15 minutes in the oven.
4. Once the squash is cooked, place it in a food processor together with the rest of the ingredients.
5. Pulse until smooth.
6. Place in individual containers.
7. Put a label and store it in the fridge.

8. Allow to warm at room temperature before heating in the microwave oven.
9. Serve with carrots or celery sticks.

Nutrition:
Calories: 109, Fat: 6 g, Carbs: 15 g, Protein: 2 g, Sugar: 3 g, Fiber: 4 g, Sodium: 14 mg, Potassium: 379 mg

153. Stir-Fried Beans and Mushrooms
Preparation Time: 15 minutes
Cooking Time: 10 minutes
Servings: 4
Ingredients:

- 1 tablespoon olive oil
- ½-pound green beans
- 4 oz. fresh mushrooms, thinly sliced
- 1 teaspoon black pepper

Directions:

1. Heat oil in the skillet over medium-high heat. Stir in green beans and mushrooms, and cook 3 to 4 minutes, until tender.
2. Transfer beans and mushrooms to a medium bowl. Toss with black pepper and serve warm.

Nutrition:
Calories: 43, Fat: 3.6 g, Sodium: 1 mg, Carbs: 2.1 g, Fiber: 0.7 g, Sugar: 1.1 g, Protein: 1.1 g, Calcium: 10 mg, Iron: 1 mg, Potassium: 56 mg, Phosphorus: 48 mg

154. Celery Salad
Preparation Time: 10 minutes
Cooking Time: 0 minutes
Servings: 4
Ingredients:

- 1 cup sliced celery
- ⅓ cup dried sweet cherries
- ⅓ cup frozen green peas, thawed
- 3 tablespoons chopped fresh basil

- 1 tablespoon chopped macadamia nuts, toasted
- 1 ½ tablespoon fat-free mayonnaise
- 1 ½ teaspoon fresh lemon juice
- ⅛ teaspoon salt
- ⅛ teaspoon ground black pepper

Directions:

1. In a medium bowl, combine the celery, cherries, peas, basil, and macadamia nuts.
2. Stir in the mayonnaise, and lemon juice.
3. Season with salt and pepper.
4. Chill before serving.

Nutrition:
Calories: 56, Fat: 3.1 g, Cholesterol: 1 mg, Sodium; 135 mg, Carbs: 5.9 g, Fiber: 1.3 g, Sugar: 1.4 g, Protein: 1.5 g, Calcium: 20 mg, Potassium: 121 mg, Phosphorus: 98 mg

155. Beans with Basil
Preparation Time: 05 minutes
Cooking Time: 05 minutes
Servings: 4
Ingredients:

- 2 teaspoons butter
- ¾ pound green beans, trimmed
- 3 green onions, chopped
- 1 clove garlic, chopped
- ⅛ teaspoon salt
- ⅛ teaspoon pepper
- 1 tablespoon chopped fresh Basil

Directions:

1. Melt the butter in a large skillet over medium heat.
2. Add the beans, green onion, and garlic.
3. Season with salt and pepper.
4. Stir-fry for 4 minutes, then remove from heat and stir in the basil leaves.

Nutrition:
Calories: 21, Fat: 1.3 g, Cholesterol: 3 mg, Sodium: 61 mg, Carbs: 2 g, Fiber: 0.7 g, Sugar: 0.8 g, Protein: 0.7 g, Calcium: 15 mg, Potassium: 58 mg, Phosphorus: 40 mg

156. Green Pea Patties
Preparation Time: 10 minutes
Cooking Time: 15 minutes
Servings: 4
Ingredients:

- ½ pound green peas
- ½ cup all-purpose flour, or as needed
- 1 egg white
- 1 tablespoon soy milk, or as needed
- 1 teaspoon baking powder
- ⅛ teaspoon salt, or to taste
- ⅛ teaspoon ground black pepper, or to taste
- 1 tablespoon olive oil, or as needed

Directions:

1. Bring a large pot of water to a boil. Cook peas in the boiling water, stirring occasionally until tender, about 5 minutes. Drain and transfer to a bowl, mash peas using a fork.
2. Mix flour, egg white, milk, baking powder, and pepper into mashed peas, adding more milk or flour until mixture holds together. Shape pea mixture into patties about ½-inch thick.
3. Heat olive oil in a skillet over medium heat, fry patties until golden, 3 to 4 minutes per side.

Nutrition:
Calories: 91, Fat: 3.5 g, Cholesterol: 28 mg, Sodium: 24 mg, Carbs: 11.7 g, Fiber: 1.1 g, Sugar: 0.8 g, Protein: 3.6 g, Calcium: 56 mg, Iron: 1 mg, Potassium: 140 mg, Phosphorus: 124 mg

157. Peas and Cauliflower
Preparation Time: 10 minutes
Cooking Time: 20 minutes
Servings: 4
Ingredients:

- 3 tablespoons olive oil
- 4 teaspoons cumin seed
- 1 teaspoon mustard seed
- 2 cups green peas
- 2 cups cauliflower florets
- ⅛ teaspoon salt
- ⅛ teaspoon pepper

Directions:

1. Heat the oil in a skillet over medium heat. Place the cumin seeds and mustard seeds in the hot oil.
2. Cook and stir until the seeds begin to pop.
3. Mix in the peas and cauliflower. Season with salt.
4. Reduce heat to low, cover, and continue cooking 15 minutes, until the vegetables are tender.

Nutrition:
Calories: 78, Fat: 4.4 g, Sodium: 87 mg, Carbs: 7.8 g, Fiber: 2.8 g, Sugar: 2.8 g, Protein: 3.1 g, Calcium: 39 mg, Iron: 2 mg, Potassium: 208 mg, Phosphorus: 148 mg

158. Mashed Peas
Preparation Time: 15 minutes
Cooking Time: 10 minutes
Servings: 4
Ingredients:

- 2 tablespoons olive oil
- 1 cup green peas
- 1 bunch fresh minutest leaves
- 1 bunch green onions, chopped
- 2 tablespoons honey
- Salt and pepper to taste

Directions:

1. Heat the olive oil in a skillet and stir the peas, minutest leaves, and green onions until the peas are hot and tender but still bright green, 7 to 10 minutes.

2. Pour the peas into a bowl, and mash until the peas are thoroughly crushed but still slightly chunky.

3. Stir in the honey, and salt and pepper, and mix until the honey is mixed well. Serve warm or cold.

Nutrition:

Calories: 83, Fat: 4.8 g, Sodium: 2 mg, Carbs: 9.6 g, Fiber: 1.5 g, Sugar: 7.2 g, Protein: 1.4 g, Calcium: 12 mg, Iron: 1 mg, Potassium: 78 mg, Phosphorus: 48 mg

159. Stuffed Zucchini Boats
Preparation Time: 15 minutes
Cooking Time: 20 minutes
Servings: 4
Ingredients:

- 2 medium zucchinis
- 4 slices white bread
- ¼ teaspoon ground sage
- 1 teaspoon onion powder
- ¼ teaspoon dried basil
- 1 teaspoon salt-free lemon pepper
- 1 teaspoon dill weed

Directions:

1. Pre-heat oven to 375 degrees F.
2. Cut zucchini in half lengthwise. Using a spoon, scoop out seeds, forming a trench in each zucchini half.
3. Place zucchini in a pot of boiling water, and boil for 3 to 5 minutes.
4. While zucchini is cooking, toast 2 slices of bread.
5. Place toast and 2 uncooked pieces of bread in a food processor to make breadcrumbs.
6. Add seasonings to breadcrumbs and mix well.
7. Add ½ cup of the zucchini cooking water and blend with a fork to get the consistency of stuffing.
8. Remove zucchini from water and place in 8 x 8" baking dish, peel side down.
9. Spoon stuffing into a trench in each zucchini half.

10. Bake for 20 minutes and serve.

Nutrition:
Calories: 42, Fat: 0.5 g, Sodium: 72 mg, Carbs: 8.5 g, Fiber: 1.4 g, Sugar: 2.3 g, Protein: 2 g, Calcium: 36 mg, Iron: 1 mg, Potassium: 283 mg, Phosphorus: 63 mg

160. Summer Squash Soup
Preparation Time: 25 minutes
Cooking Time: 35 minutes
Servings: 4
Ingredients:

- 4 tablespoons chopped onion
- 2 tablespoons olive oil
- 4 cups peeled and cubed summer squash
- 3 cups of water
- ½ teaspoon dried marjoram
- ¼ teaspoon ground black pepper
- ⅛ teaspoon ground cayenne pepper

Directions:

1. In a large saucepan, sauté onions in olive oil until tender. Add squash, water, marjoram, black pepper, and cayenne pepper. Bring to boil, cook 20 minutes, or until squash is tender.
2. Puree squash in a blender or food processor in batches until smooth.
3. Return to saucepan, and heat through. Do not allow to boil.

Nutrition:
Calories: 56, Fat: 4.8 g, Sodium: 12 mg, Carbs: 3.5 g, Fiber: 1.1 g, Sugar: 1.7 g, Protein: 1.1 g, Calcium: 19 mg, Potassium: 230 mg, Phosphorus: 150 mg

161. Sautéed Kale with Apples
Preparation Time: 15 minutes
Cooking Time: 15 minutes
Servings: 4
Ingredients:

- 1 tablespoon olive oil
- 1 onion, sliced
- 2 Red Delicious apples, cored and cut into bite-size pieces
- 2 teaspoons lemon juice
- ⅛ teaspoon of sea salt
- ⅛ teaspoon ground black pepper
- 2 cups chopped kale leaves

Directions:

1. Heat olive oil in a large skillet over medium heat, cook and stir onion until tender, about 4 minutes.
2. Add apples, lemon juice, salt, and pepper, cover skillet, and cook for about 3 minutes until apples are tender.
3. Add kale, cover, and cook until kale is tender, 4 to 5 minutes.

Nutrition:
Calories: 87, Fat: 3.7 g, Sodium: 75 mg, Carbs: 13.9 g, Fiber: 2.5 g, Sugar: 7 g, Protein: 1.5 g, Calcium: 52 mg, Iron: 1 mg, Potassium: 268 mg, Phosphorus: 110 mg

162. Creamy Mushroom Peas
Preparation Time: 1 minute
Cooking Time: 5 minutes
Servings: 4
Ingredients:

- 2 cups frozen green peas
- 2 tablespoons olive oil
- 1 cup sliced fresh mushrooms
- 1 small, chopped onion
- 1 tablespoon all-purpose flour
- ¼ teaspoon ground black pepper
- 1 pinch ground cinnamon

Directions:

1. Fill a small saucepan with one inch of water. Bring to a boil, add peas, and cook until tender, about 5 minutes. Drain and set aside.

2. Heat oil in a medium saucepan over medium heat. Add mushrooms and onions, and cook for a few minutes, or until tender. Sprinkle flour over the mushrooms, and cook for 1 minute, stirring constantly. Season with pepper and cinnamon. Cook, stirring until smooth and thick. Stir in peas and remove from heat. Let stand for 5 minutes before serving.

Nutrition:
Calories: 128, Fat: 6.1 g, Cholesterol: 15 mg, Sodium: 46 mg, Carbs: 14.3 g, Fiber: 4.4 g, Sugar: 5.2 g, Protein: 4.9 g, Calcium: 25 mg, Iron: 2 mg, Potassium: 264 mg, Phosphorus: 45 mg

163. Broccoli with Garlic Butter and Almonds
Preparation Time: 10 minutes
Cooking Time: 50 minutes
Servings: 3
Ingredients:

- 1-pound fresh broccoli, cut into bite-size pieces
- ¼ cup olive oil
- ½ tablespoon honey
- 1-½ tablespoons soy sauce
- ¼ teaspoon ground black pepper
- 2 cloves garlic, minced
- ¼ cup chopped almonds

Directions:

1. Place the broccoli into a large pot with about 1 inch of water in the bottom. Drain, and arrange broccoli on a Servings: platter.
2. While the broccoli is cooking, heat the oil in a small skillet over medium heat. Mix in the honey, soy sauce, pepper, and garlic. Bring to a boil, then remove from the heat. Mix in the almonds and pour the sauce over the broccoli. Serve immediately.

Nutrition:
Calories: 177, Sodium: 234 mg, Protein: 2.9 g, Potassium: 13 mg, Phosphorus: 67 mg

164. Eggplant French Fries
Preparation Time: 10 minutes

Cooking Time: 50 minutes
Servings: 4
Ingredients:

- 1 medium eggplant
- 1 cup soy milk
- 2 large eggs
- ¼ cup cornstarch
- ¼ cup dry unseasoned breadcrumbs
- ½ cup olive oil
- ½ tablespoon pepper

Directions:

1. Peel and slice eggplant into ¾-inch sticks, 4-inch long. Rinse and pat dry.
2. In a medium bowl, mix milk and eggs until well blended.
3. Heat oil in a frying pan on high heat.
4. Place in oil, flipping regularly, and fry 3 minutes or until golden brown.
5. Drain on paper towels and serve immediately.

Nutrition:
Calories: 269, Sodium: 112 mg, Protein: 5.5 g, Potassium: 270 mg, Phosphorus: 167 mg

165. Thai Tofu Broth
Preparation Time: 5 minutes
Cooking Time: 15 minutes
Servings: 4
Ingredients:

- 1 cup rice noodles
- ½ sliced onion
- 6 oz. drained, pressed, and cubed tofu
- ¼ cup sliced scallions
- ½ cup water
- ½ cup canned water chestnuts
- ½ cup rice milk
- 1 tbsp. lime juice

- 1 tbsp. coconut oil
- ½ finely sliced chili
- 1 cup snow peas

Directions:

1. Heat the oil in a wok on high heat and then sauté the tofu until brown on each side.
2. Add the onion and sauté for 2-3 minutes. Add the rice milk and water to the wok until bubbling.
3. Lower to medium heat and add the noodles, chili, and water chestnuts.
4. Allow to simmer for 10-15 minutes and then add the sugar snap peas for 5 minutes. Serve with a sprinkle of scallions.

Nutrition:
Calories: 304, Protein: 9 g, Carbs: 38 g, Fat: 13 g, Sodium: 36 mg, Potassium: 114 mg, Phosphorus: 101 mg

Snacks Recipes

166. Candied Macadamia Nuts
Preparation Time: 10 Minutes
Cooking Time: 15 Minutes
Servings: 2
Ingredients:
- 2 cups macadamia nuts
- 1 tablespoon extra-virgin olive oil
- 2 tablespoons honey

Directions:

1. In a bowl, toss together all Ingredients: and spread into a baking dish. Bake at 350°F for about 15 minutes or until browned.
2. Remove from oven and let cool before serving.

Nutrition: Calories: 602, Fat: 58.9 g, Carbs: 23.3 g, Fiber: 5.9 g, Protein: 5.7 g, Sodium: 236 mg, Sugars: 20.1 g
167. Peanut Butter Fudge

Preparation Time: 5 Minutes
Cooking Time: 2 Minutes
Servings: 12
Ingredients:
* ¼ cup vanilla almond milk
* 1 cup coconut oil
* 1 cup peanut butter

Optional Topping:
* 2 tablespoons melted coconut oil
* ¼ cup unsweetened cocoa powder
* 2 tablespoons raw honey

Directions:

1. Melt coconut oil and peanut butter over low heat, transfer to a blender along with the remaining Ingredients: and blend until very smooth.
2. Pour the mixture into a loaf pan lined with parchment paper. Whisk the topping Ingredients: in a bowl and drizzle over the fudge. Freeze until firm and serve.

Nutrition:
Calories: 287, Fat: 29.7 g, Carbs: 4 g, Fiber: 1.7 g, Sugars: 0.7 g, Protein: 5.4 g, Sodium: 4 mg

168. Apple & Strawberry Snack
Preparation Time: 5 Minutes
Cooking Time: 2 Minutes
Servings: 1
Ingredients:
* ½ apple, cored and sliced
* 2-3 strawberries
* dash of ground cinnamon
* 2-3 drops stevia 2-3 drops

Directions:

1. In a bowl, mix strawberries and apples and sprinkle with stevia and cinnamon, microwave for about 1-2 minutes. Serve warm.

Nutrition:

Calories: 145, Fat: 0.8 g, Carbs: 34.2 g, Fiber: 7.8 g, Sugars: 24.4 g, Protein: 1.6 g, Sodium: 11 mg

169. Cinnamon Applesauce
Preparation Time: 10 Minutes
Cooking Time: 0 Minutes
Servings: 1
Ingredients:
- 1 apple
- Powdered stevia
- ½ teaspoon cinnamon
- Pinch of nutmeg

Directions:

1. Puree apple in a food processor along with stevia and cinnamon.
2. Chill before serving.

Nutrition:
Calories: 146, Fat: 0.7 g, Carbs: 36.4 g, Fiber: 6.8 g, Sugars: 26.4 g, Protein: 1.6 g, Sodium: 10 mg

170. Cinnamon Apple Chips
Preparation Time: 10 Minutes
Cooking Time: 15 Minutes
Servings: 1
Ingredients:
- 1 apple, sliced thinly
- Dash of cinnamon
- Stevia

Directions:

1. Coat apple slices with cinnamon and stevia and bake at 325°F for about 15 minutes or until tender and crispy.

Nutrition:
Calories: 146, Fat: 0.7 g, Carbs: 36.4 g, Fiber: 6.8 g, Sugars: 26.4 g, Protein: 1.6 g, Sodium: 10 mg

171. Lemon Pops
Preparation Time: 5 Minutes
Cooking Time: 0 Minutes

Servings: 1
Ingredients:
- 4 tablespoons fresh lemon juice
- Powdered stevia

Directions:

1. Mix orange or lemon juice and stevia and pour into molds, freeze until firm.

Nutrition:
Sodium: 10 mg

172. Strawberry Sorbet
Preparation Time: 5 Minutes
Cooking Time: 0 Minutes
Servings: 1
Ingredients:
- 4-6 medium strawberries
- 2 tablespoons fresh lemon juice
- ½ teaspoon vanilla powder
- Flavored stevia
- Ice cubes
- ¼ cup water

Directions:

1. In a blender, blend all Ingredients: until very smooth, pour into molds and freeze until firm.

Nutrition:
Calories: 26, Fat: 0.3 g, Carbs: 4.7 g, Fiber: 2.7 g, Sugars: 1.7 g, Protein: 1.6 g, Sodium: 9 mg

173. Tasty Candied Pecans
Preparation Time: 15 Minutes
Cooking Time: 15 Minutes
Servings: 4
Ingredients:
- ½ cup pecans
- 2 tablespoons maple syrup
- 1 tablespoon extra-virgin olive oil
- ½ teaspoon of sea salt

Directions:

1. In a bowl, toss together all Ingredients: and spread into a baking dish. Bake at 350°F for about 15 minutes.
2. Remove from oven and let cool before serving.

Nutrition:
Calories: 315, Fat: 30.3 g, Carbs: 12.1 g, Fiber: 4 g, Protein: 4 g, Sodium: 235 mg, Sugars: 7.3 g

174. Easy No-Bake Coconut Cookies
Preparation Time: 2 Minutes
Cooking Time: 10 Minutes
Servings: 20
Ingredients:
- 3 cups finely shredded coconut flakes
- 1 cup melted coconut oil
- 1 teaspoon liquid stevia

Directions:

1. Combine all ingredients in a large bowl, stir until well blended.
2. Form the mixture into small balls and arrange them on a paper-lined baking tray.
3. Press each cookie down with a fork and refrigerate until firm. Enjoy!

Nutrition:
Calories: 99, Fat: 10 g, Carbs: 2 g, Fiber: 2 g, Protein: 3 g, Sodium: 7 mg

175. Roasted Chili-Vinegar Peanuts
Preparation Time: 10 Minutes
Cooking Time: 0 Minutes
Servings: 4
Ingredients:
- 1 tablespoon coconut oil
- 2 cups raw peanuts, unsalted
- 2 teaspoon of sea salt
- 2 tablespoon apple cider vinegar
- 1 teaspoon chili powder
- 1 teaspoon fresh lime zest

Directions:

1. Preheat oven to 350°F.
2. In a large bowl, toss together coconut oil, peanuts, and salt until well coated.
3. Transfer to a rimmed baking sheet and roast in the oven for about 15 minutes or until fragrant.
4. Transfer the roasted peanuts to a bowl and add vinegar, chili powder, and lime zest.
5. Toss to coat well and serve.

Nutrition:
Calories: 447, Fat: 39.5g, Carbs: 12.3 g, Fiber: 6.5 g, Sugars: 3 g, Protein: 18.9 g, Sodium: 956 mg

176. Healthy Spiced Nuts
Preparation Time: 10 Minutes
Cooking Time: 10 Minutes
Servings: 4
Ingredients:
- 1 tbsp. extra virgin olive oil
- ¼ cup walnuts
- ¼ cup pecans
- ¼ cup almonds
- ½ tsp. sea salt
- ½ tsp. pepper
- ½ tsp. cumin
- 1 tsp. chili powder

Directions:

1. Put the nuts in a skillet set over medium heat and toast until lightly browned.
2. In the meantime, prepare the spice mixture, combine black pepper, cumin, chili, and salt in a bowl.
3. Coat the toasted nuts with extra virgin olive oil and sprinkle with the spice mixture to serve.

Nutrition:
Calories: 221, Fat: 22 g, Carbs: 4.8 g, Fiber: 3.2 g, Protein: 4.9 g, Sodium: 241 mg

177. Roasted Asparagus
Preparation Time: 5 Minutes

Cooking Time: 10 Minutes
Servings: 4
Ingredients:
- 1 tbsp. extra virgin olive oil
- 1-pound fresh asparagus
- 1 medium lemon, zested
- ½ tsp. freshly grated nutmeg
- ½ tsp. black pepper

Directions:

1. Preheat your oven to 500°F.
2. Arrange asparagus on an aluminum foil and drizzle with extra virgin olive oil, toss until well coated.
3. Spread the asparagus in a single layer and fold the edges of foil to make a tray.
4. Roast the asparagus in the oven for about 5 minutes, toss, and continue roasting for 5 minutes more or until browned.
5. Sprinkle the roasted asparagus with nutmeg, salt, zest, and pepper to serve.

Nutrition:
Calories: 55, Fat: 3.8 g, Carbs: 4.7 g, Fiber: 2.5 g, Protein: 2.5 g, Sodium: 293 mg

178. Warm Lemon Rosemary Olives
Preparation Time: 5 Minutes
Cooking Time: 20 Minutes
Servings: 12 Servings
Ingredients:
- 1 teaspoon extra-virgin olive oil
- 1 teaspoon grated lemon peel
- 1 teaspoon crushed red pepper flakes
- 2 sprigs fresh rosemary
- 3 cups mixed olives
- Lemon twists, optional

Directions:

1. Preheat your oven to 400°F. Place pepper flakes, rosemary, olives, and grated lemon peel onto a large sheet of foil, drizzle

with oil and fold the foil. Pinch the edges of the sheet to tightly seal.

2. Bake in the preheated oven for about 30 minutes. Remove from the sheet and place the mixture in the serving dish. Serve warm garnished with lemon twists.

Nutrition:
Calories: 43, Fat: 4 g, Carbs: 2.2 g, Fiber: 1.1 g, Protein: 0.3 g, Sodium: 293 mg,

179. Low-Fat Mango Salsa
Preparation Time: 20 Minutes
Cooking Time: 0 Minutes
Servings: 4
Ingredients:
- 1 cup cucumber, chopped
- 2 cups mango, diced
- ½ cup cilantro, minced
- 2 tablespoons fresh lime juice
- 1 tablespoon scallions, minced
- ¼ teaspoon chipotle powder
- ¼ teaspoon of sea salt

Directions:

1. Mix all ingredients in a bowl and serve or refrigerate.

Nutrition:
Calories: 155, Fat: 0.6 g, Carbs: 38.2 g, Fiber: 4.1 g, Protein: 1.4 g, Sodium: 123 mg, Sugars: 31.9 g

180. Vinegar & Salt Kale Chips
Preparation Time: 10 Minutes
Cooking Time: 12 Minutes
Servings: 2
Ingredients:
- 1 head kale, chopped
- 1 teaspoon extra virgin olive oil
- 1 tablespoon apple cider vinegar
- ½ teaspoon of sea salt

Directions:

1. Place kale in a bowl and drizzle with vinegar and extra virgin olive oil, sprinkle with salt and massage the Ingredients: with hands.
2. Spread the kale out onto two paper-lined baking sheets and bake at 375°F for about 12 minutes or until crispy.
3. Let cool for about 10 minutes before serving.

Nutrition:
Calories: 152, Fat: 8.2 g, Carbs: 15.2 g, Fiber: 2 g, Protein: 4 g, Sodium: 1066 mg

181. Carrot and Parsnips French Fries
Preparation Time: 15 Minutes
Cooking Time: 20 Minutes
Servings: 2
Ingredients:
- 6 large carrots
- 6 large parsnips
- 2 tablespoons extra virgin olive oil
- ½ teaspoon of sea salt

Directions:

1. Chop the carrots and parsnips into 2-inch sections and then cut each section into thin sticks.
2. Toss together the carrots and parsnip sticks with extra virgin olive oil and salt in a bowl and spread into a baking sheet lined with parchment paper.
3. Bake the sticks at 425° for about 20 minutes or until browned.

Nutrition:
Calories: 209, Fat: 14 g, Carbs: 21.2 g, Fiber: 5.3 g, Protein: 1.8 g, Sodium: 617 mg, Sugars: 10.6 g

182. Cinnamon Tortilla Chips
Preparation Time: 15 minutes
Cooking Time: 10 minutes
Servings: 6
Ingredients:
- 2 tsp Granulated sugar
- ½ tsp Ground cinnamon
- Pinch ground nutmeg

- 3 (6-inch) Flour tortillas
- Cooking spray

Directions:

1. Preheat the oven to 350°F.
2. Line a baking sheet with parchment paper.
3. In a small bowl, stir together the sugar, cinnamon, and nutmeg.
4. Lay the tortillas on a clean work surface and spray both sides of each lightly with cooking spray.
5. Sprinkle the cinnamon sugar evenly over both sides of each tortilla.
6. Cut the tortillas into 16 wedges each and place them on the baking sheet.
7. Bake the tortilla wedges, turning once, for about 10 minutes or until crisp.
8. Cool the chips
9. Serve.

Nutrition:
Calories: 51, Fat: 1 g, Carbs: 9 g, Phosphorus: 29 mg, Potassium: 24 mg, Protein: 1 g

183. Sweet and Spicy Kettle Corn
Preparation Time: 1 minute
Cooking Time: 5 minutes
Servings: 8
Ingredients:
- 3 tbsp. Olive oil
- 1 cup Popcorn kernels
- ½ cup Brown sugar
- Pinch cayenne pepper

Directions:

1. Place a large pot with a lid over medium heat and add the olive oil with a few popcorn kernels.
2. Shake the pot lightly until the popcorn kernels pop. Add the rest of the kernels and sugar to the pot.
3. Pop the kernels with the lid on the pot, constantly shaking, until they are popped.

4. Remove the pot from the heat and transfer the popcorn to a large bowl.
5. Toss the popcorn with the cayenne pepper and serve.

Nutrition:
Calories: 186, Fat: 6 g, Carbs: 30 g, Phosphorus: 85 mg, Potassium: 90 mg, Sodium: 5 mg, Protein: 3 g

184. Meringue Cookies
Preparation Time: 30 minutes
Cooking Time: 30 minutes
Servings: 24
Ingredients:
- 4 Egg whites
- 1 cup Granulated sugar
- 1 tsp. Pure vanilla extract
- 1 tsp. Almond extract

Directions:

1. Preheat the oven to 300°F.
2. Line 2 baking sheets with parchment paper. Set aside.
3. Beat the egg whites until soft peaks form.
4. Add the granulated sugar 1 tbsp. at a time. Beat well to mix after each addition. The meringue should be thick and glossy.
5. Beat in the vanilla extract and almond extract.
6. Using a tbsp., drop the meringue batter onto the baking sheets, spacing the cookies evenly.
7. Bake the cookies for 30 minutes, or until they are crisp.
8. Remove the cookies from the oven and let them cool on wire racks.
9. Serve.

Nutrition:
Calories: 36, Carbs: 8 g, Phosphorus: 1 mg, Potassium: 10 mg, Sodium: 9 mg, Protein: 1 g

185. Corn Bread
Preparation Time: 10 minutes
Cooking Time: 20 minutes
Servings: 10
Ingredients:

- Cooking spray for greasing the baking dish
- 1 ¼ cups Yellow cornmeal
- ¾ cup All-purpose flour
- 1 tbsp. Baking soda substitute
- ½ cup Granulated sugar
- 2 Eggs
- 1 cup Unsweetened, unfortified rice milk
- 2 tbsp. Olive oil

Directions:

1. Preheat the oven to 425°F.
2. Lightly spray an 8-by-8-inch baking dish with cooking spray. Set aside.
3. In a medium bowl, stir together the cornmeal, flour, baking soda substitute, and sugar.
4. In a small bowl, whisk together the eggs, rice milk, and olive oil until blended.
5. Add the wet ingredients to the dry ingredients and stir until well combined.
6. Pour the batter into the baking dish and bake for 20 minutes or until golden and cooked through.
7. Serve warm.

Nutrition:
Calories: 198, Fat: 5 g, Carbs: 34 g, Phosphorus: 88 mg, Potassium: 94 mg, Sodium: 25 mg, Protein: 4 g

186. Cucumber-Wrapped Vegetable Rolls
Preparation Time: 30 minutes
Cooking Time: 0 minutes
Servings: 8
Ingredients:
- ½ cup Finely shredded red cabbage
- ½ cup Grated carrot
- ¼ cup Julienne red bell pepper
- ¼ cup Julienned scallion, both green and white parts
- ¼ cup Chopped cilantro
- 1 tbsp. Olive oil
- ¼ tsp. ground cumin
- ¼ tsp. Freshly ground black pepper

- 1 English cucumber, sliced into very thin strips

Directions:

1. In a bowl, toss together the black pepper, cumin, olive oil, cilantro, scallion, red pepper, carrot, and cabbage. Mix well.
2. Evenly divide the vegetable filling among the cucumber strips, placing the filling close to one end of the strip.
3. Roll up the cucumber strips around the filling and secure with a wooden pick.
4. Repeat with each cucumber strip.

Nutrition:
Calories: 26, Fat: 2 g, Carbs: 3 g, Phosphorus: 14 mg, Potassium: 95 mg, Sodium: 7 mg

187. Chicken-Vegetable Kebabs
Preparation Time: 15 minutes
Cooking Time: 12 minutes
Servings: 4
Ingredients:
- 2 tbsp. Olive oil
- 2 tbsp. Freshly squeezed lemon juice
- ½ tsp Minced garlic
- ½ tsp Chopped fresh thyme
- 4 ounces Boneless, skinless chicken breast, cut into 8 pieces
- 1Small summer squash, cut into 8 pieces
- ½Medium onion, cut into 8 pieces

Directions:

1. Stir together the olive oil, lemon juice, garlic, and thyme in a bowl.
2. Add the chicken to the bowl and stir to coat.
3. Cover the bowl with plastic wrap and place the chicken in the refrigerator to marinate for 1 hour.
4. Thread the squash, onion, and chicken pieces onto 4 large skewers, evenly dividing the vegetable and meat among the skewers.
5. Heat a barbecue to medium and grill the skewers, turning at least 2 times, for 10 to 12 minutes or until the chicken is cooked through.

Nutrition:
Calories: 106, Fat: 8 g, Carbs: 3 g, Phosphorus: 77 mg, Potassium: 199 mg, Sodium: 14 mg, Protein: 7 g

188. Chicken Lettuce Wraps
Preparation Time: 30 minutes
Cooking Time: 0 minutes
Servings: 8
Ingredients:
- 6 ounces Cooked chicken breast, minced
- 1 Scallion, both green and white parts, chopped
- ½ Red apple, cored and chopped
- ½ cup Bean sprouts
- ¼ English cucumber, chopped
- Juice of 1 lime
- Zest of 1 lime
- 2 tbsp. Chopped fresh cilantro
- ½ tsp Chinese five-spice powder
- 8 Boston lettuce leaves

Directions:

1. In a bowl, mix the scallions, chicken, apple, cucumber, bean sprouts, lime juice, lime zest, cilantro, and five-spice powder.
2. Spoon the chicken mixture evenly among the 8 lettuce leaves.
3. Wrap the lettuce around the chicken mixture and serve.

Nutrition:
Calories: 51, Fat: 2 g, Carbs: 2 g, Phosphorus: 56 mg, Potassium: 110 mg, Sodium: 16 mg, Protein: 7 g

189. Antojitos
Preparation Time: 20 minutes
Cooking Time: 0 minutes
Servings: 8
Ingredients:
- 6 ounces plain cream cheese
- ½ Jalapeno pepper, finely chopped
- ½ Scallion, green part only, chopped
- ¼ cup red bell pepper, finely chopped
- ½ tsp. ground cumin
- ½ tsp. Ground coriander

- ½ tsp Chili powder
- 3 (8-inch) flour tortillas

Directions:

1. In a bowl, mix the jalapeno pepper, cream cheese, scallion, red bell pepper, cumin, coriander, and chili powder until well blended.
2. Divide the cream cheese mixture evenly among the 3 tortillas, spreading the cheese in a thin layer and leaving a ¼ inch edge all the way around.
3. Roll the tortillas like a jelly roll and wrap each tightly in plastic wrap.
4. Refrigerate the rolls for about 1 hour or until they are set.
5. Cut the rolls and serve.

Nutrition:
Calories: 110, Fat: 8 g, Carbs: 7 g, Phosphorus: 47 mg, Potassium: 72 mg, Sodium: 215 mg, Protein: 2 g

190. Roasted Onion Garlic Dip
Preparation Time: 15 minutes
Cooking Time: 1 hour
Servings: 6
Ingredients:
- 1 sweet onion, peeled and cut into eights
- 8 cloves Garlic
- 2 tsp Olive oil
- ½ cup light sour cream
- 1 tbsp. Fresh lemon juice
- 1 tbsp. Chopped fresh parsley
- 1 tsp. Chopped fresh thyme
- Ground black pepper

Directions:

1. Preheat the oven to 425°F.
2. Toss the onion and garlic in a bowl with olive oil.
3. Transfer the onion and garlic to a piece of aluminum foil and wrap the vegetables loosely in a packet.
4. Place the foil packet on a small baking sheet and place the sheet in the oven.

5. Roast the vegetables for 50 minutes to 1 hour, or until they are very fragrant and golden.
6. Remove the packet from the oven and allow it to cool for 15 minutes.
7. In a bowl, stir together the lemon juice, sour cream, parsley, thyme, and black pepper.
8. Open the foil packet carefully and transfer the vegetables to a cutting board.
9. Chop the vegetables and add them to the sour cream mixture. Stir to combine.
10. Cover the dip and chill in the refrigerator for 1 hour.
11. Serve.

Nutrition:
Calories: 44, Fat: 3 g, Carbs: 5 g, Phosphorus: 22 mg, Potassium: 79 mg, Sodium: 10 mg, Protein: 1 g

191. Cheese-Herb Dip
Preparation Time: 20 minutes
Cooking Time: 0 minutes
Servings: 8
Ingredients:
• 1 cup Cream cheese
• ½ cup Unsweetened rice milk
• ½ Scallion, green part only, chopped
• 1 tbsp. Chopped fresh parsley
• 1 tbsp. Chopped fresh basil
• 1 tbsp. Lemon juice
• 1 tsp. Minced garlic
• ½ tsp. Chopped fresh thyme
• ¼ tsp. Ground black pepper

Directions:

1. In a bowl, mix the milk, cream cheese, parsley, scallion, basil, lemon juice, garlic, thyme, and pepper until well combined.
2. Store and use.

Nutrition:
Calories: 108, Fat: 10 g, Carbs: 3 g, Phosphorus: 40 mg, Potassium: 52 mg, Sodium: 112 mg, Protein: 2 g

192. Baba Ghanoush
Preparation Time: 20 minutes
Cooking Time: 30 minutes
Servings: 6
Ingredients:
- 1 Eggplant, halved and scored with a crosshatch pattern on the cut sides
- 1 tbsp. Olive oil, plus extra for brushing
- 1 sweet onion, peeled and diced
- 2 cloves garlic, halved
- 1 tsp. ground cumin
- 1 tsp. Ground coriander
- 1 tbsp. Lemon juice
- Freshly ground black pepper

Directions:

1. Preheat the oven to 400°F.
2. Line 2 baking sheets with parchment paper.
3. Brush the eggplant halves with olive oil and place them, cut side down, on 1 baking sheet.
4. In a small bowl, mix the onion, garlic, 1 tbsp. olive oil, cumin, and coriander.
5. Spread the seasoned onions on the other baking sheet.
6. Place both baking sheets in the oven and roast the onions for about 20 minutes and the eggplant for 30 minutes, or until softened and browned.
7. Remove the vegetables from the oven and scrape the eggplant flesh into a bowl.
8. Transfer the onions and garlic to a cutting board and chop coarsely, add to the eggplant.
9. Stir in the lemon juice and pepper.
10. Serve warm or chilled.

Nutrition:
Calories: 45, Fat: 2 g, Carbs: 6 g, Phosphorus: 23 mg, Potassium: 195 mg, Sodium: 3 mg, Protein: 1 g

193. Spicy Kale Chips
Preparation Time: 20 minutes
Cooking Time: 25 minutes

Servings: 6
Ingredients:
- 2 cups Kale
- 2 tsp. Olive oil
- ¼ tsp. Chili powder
- Pinch cayenne pepper

Directions:

1. Preheat the oven to 300°F.
2. Line 2 baking sheets with parchment paper, set aside.
3. Remove the stems from the kale and tear the leaves into 2-inch pieces.
4. Wash the kale and dry it completely.
5. Transfer the kale to a large bowl and drizzle with olive oil.
6. Use your hands to toss the kale with oil, taking care to coat each leaf evenly.
7. Season the kale with chili powder and cayenne pepper and toss to combine thoroughly.
8. Spread the seasoned kale in a single layer on each baking sheet. Do not overlap the leaves.
9. Bake the kale, rotating the pans once, for 20 to 25 minutes until it is crisp and dry.
10. Remove the trays from the oven and allow the chips to cool on the trays for 5 minutes.
11. Serve.

Nutrition:
Calories: 24, Fat: 2 g, Carbs: 2 g, Phosphorus: 21 mg, Potassium: 111 mg, Sodium: 13 mg, Protein: 1 g

194. Fluffy Fruit Dip
Preparation Time: 5 minutes
Cooking Time: 10 minutes
Servings: 8
Ingredients:

- 7 oz. marshmallow cream
- 1 tbsp. dried orange peel
- 8 oz. low-fat, plain cream cheese

Directions:

1. Mix all ingredients until smooth.

Nutrition:
Calories 183, Carbs 22 g, Phosphorus 31 mg, Potassium 36 mg, Protein 2 g, Sodium 104 mg

195. Perfect Pretzels
Preparation Time: 30 minutes
Cooking Time: 60 minutes
Servings: 32
Ingredients:

- 32 oz. unsalted pretzels
- 1 cup canola oil
- 3 tsp garlic powder
- 3 tsp dried dill weed
- 2 tbsp. low-sodium ranch salad dressing and seasoning mix

Directions:

1. Preheat oven to 175°F.
2. Pack pretzels out flat onto two 18-inch x 13-inch baking sheets. Combine the dill and garlic powder and split the seasonings into two. To one half of the seasoning add the dry salad dressing mix and ¾ cup canola oil.
3. Pour the mixture evenly over the pretzels, coating evenly. Bake for 1 hour, flipping the pretzels every 15 minutes.
4. Remove the pretzels from the oven and allow to cool and toss with the remaining seasoning mix.

Nutrition:
Calories: 184, Carbs: 22 g, Phosphorus: 28 mg, Potassium: 43 mg, Protein: 2 g, Sodium: 60 mg

196. BBQ Meatballs
Preparation Time: 15 minutes
Cooking Time: 25 minutes
Servings: 24
Ingredients:

- 3 pounds' lean ground beef
- ½ cup finely chopped onion
- 2 large beaten eggs
- 1 cup uncooked oatmeal
- ½ cup unenriched rice milk or milk alternative
- 1 tbsp. dried thyme
- 1 tsp dried oregano
- ½ tsp pepper
- 1 cup low-sodium BBQ sauce
- ⅓ cup water

Directions:

1. Preheat oven to 375°F.
2. In a large bowl, mix all ingredients except low-sodium BBQ sauce and water. The best tools for this job are your hands. Roll mixture into one-inch balls and place on a baking sheet.
3. Bake for 15 minutes until meatballs are cooked through.
4. In a warming dish, mix low-sodium BBQ sauce and water and stand over a low-temperature setting. Add meatballs to the dish and stir. Cover and serve.

Nutrition:
Calories: 176, Carbs: 6 g, Phosphorus: 107 mg, Potassium: 208 mg, Protein: 11 g, Sodium: 180 mg

197. Spicy Chicken Wings
Preparation Time: 15 minutes
Cooking Time: 30 minutes
Servings: 4
Ingredients:

- 1-pound fresh chicken wings
- ¼ cup honey
- 1 ½ tbsp. diced chipotle peppers
- ¼ cup unsalted butter
- 1 tsp black pepper
- 1 tbsp. chopped chives
- Oil for greasing the tray

Directions:

1. Preheat oven to 400°F. Arrange wings on a large baking sheet.
2. Bake for 20 minutes, turning halfway through the cooking time or until crispy on the outside.
3. In a large bowl, combine the remaining ingredients with a rubber spatula.
4. Remove the wings from the oven and toss in the sauce until evenly coated. Transfer to a large platter and serve.

Nutrition:
Calories: 384, Carbs: 18 g, Phosphorus: 146 mg, Potassium: 266 mg, Protein: 20 g, Sodium: 99 mg

198. Blueberry Protein Bars
Preparation Time: 15 minutes + 60 minutes' chill
Cooking Time: 10 minutes
Servings: 12
Ingredients:

- 2 ½ cups rolled oats
- ½ cup honey
- ½ cup almonds
- ½ cup flaxseeds
- ½ cup peanut butter
- 1 cup dried blueberries

Directions:

1. In a 350°F oven, toast oats by scattering on a baking sheet and bake for 10 minutes or until golden.
2. Remove from oven and combine with all ingredients. Mix well.
3. Lightly grease a 9-inch square pan and press mix down into the pan. Wrap and refrigerate for at least one hour.
4. Cut protein bars into 12 squares.

Nutrition:
Calories: 283, Carbs: 39 g, Phosphorus: 177 mg, Potassium: 258 mg, Protein: 7 g, Sodium: 49 mg

199. Delicious Deviled Eggs

Preparation Time: 10 minutes
Cooking Time: 15 minutes
Servings: 4
Ingredients:

- 4 large hard-boiled, de-shelled eggs
- 1 tbsp. finely chopped onion
- ½ tsp cider vinegar
- 2 tsp mayonnaise
- ¼ tsp black pepper
- ½ tsp mustard powder
- Dash of paprika

Directions:

1. Slice eggs down the middle and carefully remove egg yolk. Place egg whites flat onto a large platter and yolks into a small bowl.
2. Add dry mustard, vinegar, pepper, and onion to bowl with yolks and mash together.
3. Fill egg whites with yolk mixture and sprinkle with paprika.

Nutrition:
Calories: 98, Carbs: 2 g, Phosphorus: 90 mg, Potassium: 73 mg, Protein: 6 g, Sodium: 124 mg

200. Herb Biscuits
Preparation Time: 10 minutes
Cooking Time: 10 minutes
Servings: 12
Ingredients:

- 1 ¾ cups all-purpose flour
- ⅔ cup skim milk or milk alternative
- 3 tbsp. fresh or dried chives
- 3 tbsp. fresh or dried parsley
- ¼ cup mayonnaise
- 1 tsp cream of tartar
- ½ tsp baking soda
- Non-stick cooking spray

Directions:

1. Preheat oven to 400°F. Prepare a baking tray by spraying with non-stick spray.
2. Mix flour, baking soda, and cream of tartar in a large bowl. Add mayonnaise and blend with a fork until consistency is coarse.
3. Mix milk and herbs in a separate dish and add to the flour. Stir until well-mixed.
4. Heap tablespoon measures of dough onto the baking tray. Bake for 10 minutes.

Nutrition:
Calories: 109, Carbs: 15 g, Phosphorus: 34 mg, Potassium: 85 mg, Protein: 3 g, Sodium: 88 mg

201. Chickpea Eggplant Bites
Preparation Time: 30 minutes
Cooking Time: 50 minutes
Servings: 20
Ingredients:

- 14 oz. canned chickpeas
- 3 large eggplants, halved
- 2 tbsp. chickpea flour
- 3 tbsp. polenta
- 2 tsp cumin seeds
- 2 tsp cilantro
- 2 large garlic cloves, peeled
- ½ lemon zested and juice
- Cooking spray oil

Directions:

1. Heat oven to 400°F. In a large roasting tin, place eggplant halves cut side up and spray generously with oil. Add garlic, cumin, and cilantro. Roast for 40 minutes until eggplant is tender. Allow to cool slightly. Turn oven down to 350°F.
2. Scoop the eggplant flesh into a bowl and discard the skins. Scrape spices from the roasting pan into a bowl. Roughly mash with chickpeas, flour lemon juice, and zest.

3. Line a baking tray with parchment paper and shape the mixture into 20 balls, placing them on the baking tray and in the refrigerator for 30 minutes.

4. When balls are chilled, remove from refrigerator and roll in polenta, return to tray, and spray each with a little oil. Roast for 20 minutes until crisp and golden.

Nutrition:

Calories: 72, Carbs: 18 g, Phosphorus: 36 mg, Potassium: 162 mg, Protein: 3 g, Sodium: 63 mg

202. Roasted Red Pepper Dip
Preparation Time: 10 minutes
Cooking Time: 10 minutes
Servings: 4
Ingredients:

- 1 cup red peppers
- 1 clove garlic
- 1 tsp. lemon juice
- 1 tbsp. olive oil
- 1 tsp. cumin

Directions:

1. Preheat oven to 350°F. Slice peppers in half and clean. Lay cut side up on a roasting tray and spray with a very small amount of oil. Roast for 10 minutes or until peppers are tender. Remove from oven and allow to cool.

2. Blend roasted peppers and all other ingredients in a food processor until smooth.

Nutrition:

Calories: 84, Carbs: 3 g, Phosphorus: 13 mg, Potassium: 89 mg, Protein: 0.5 g, Sodium: 9 mg

203. Curried Crab Cakes
Preparation Time: 10 minutes
Cooking Time: 15 minutes
Servings: 8
Ingredients:

- 4 oz. crab meat
- ¼ cup white breadcrumbs
- ¼ cup finely chopped red pepper
- 1 finely chopped green onion
- ½ cup finely chopped parsley
- 1 clove crushed garlic
- 1 egg
- 1 tsp lemon juice
- 1 tbsp. curry powder
- Black pepper to taste
- Vegetable oil

Directions:

1. Mix all ingredients in a large bowl. Your hands are the best tools for this. Split the mixture into eight portions and squeeze all the excess liquid out of each portion. Form crab cakes with your hands.
2. Over medium-high heat coat the bottom of a frying pan with vegetable oil, and let it warm up. Fry crab cakes for two minutes on each side or until golden brown.

Nutrition:
Calories: 75, Carbs: 4 g, Phosphorus: 60 mg, Potassium: 116 mg, Protein: 5 g, Sodium: 88 mg

204. Falafel
Preparation Time: 30 minutes (soak chickpeas overnight)
Cooking Time: 15 minutes
Servings: 8
Ingredients:

- 1 pound dried chickpeas
- 2 green onions
- 2 cups white onion
- ½ cup parsley
- 4 cloves garlic
- ¼ cup lemon juice
- 1 ½ tbsp. flour
- ¾ tsp salt

- 1 tsp cilantro
- 1 tbsp. cumin
- ¼ tsp black pepper
- ¼ tsp cayenne pepper
- 2 tbsp. peanut oil

Directions:

1. Cover chickpeas in water in a large pot and soak overnight at room temperature.
2. Finely chop the white onion, green onions, parsley, and garlic. Drain and rinse the chickpeas. Place in a food processor with onions, parsley, garlic, lemon juice, cilantro, black pepper, cumin, and cayenne pepper.
3. Pulse in a food processor until the mixture has a coarse to a pasty consistency. Blend with a fork and remove any large pieces of chickpeas.
4. Refrigerate the mixture for two hours. During this time, preheat the oven to 400°F. Spray a muffin tin with cooking spray.
5. Use a scoop or roll mixture into 24 balls and place in a muffin tin. Bake for 7 minutes. Remove, turn falafel over, and then bake 7 minutes longer.

Nutrition:
Calories: 278, Carbs: 43 g, Phosphorus: 170 mg, Potassium: 548 mg, Protein: 13 g, Sodium: 239 mg

205. Vegetarian Spring Rolls
Preparation Time: 40 minutes
Cooking Time: 0 minutes
Servings: 3
Ingredients:

- 12 rice wrappers for spring rolls
- 16 oz. firm tofu
- 12 leaves lettuce
- 2 medium carrots
- ½ medium red onion
- ½ tbsp. ground cumin

- ½ tbsp. granulated garlic
- ¼ tsp sea salt
- ½ tsp black pepper
- 1 tbsp. olive oil

Directions:

1. Wash and dry the lettuce and cut each leaf in half lengthwise. Cut carrots julienne style. Slice onion. Set aside.
2. Boil 6 cups of water and set aside to soak the rice wrappers in later.
3. Drain and pat dry the tofu. Slice it into 12 4-inch pieces. Spread the tofu on a plate and season with cumin, granulated garlic, sea salt, and black pepper.
4. Heat olive oil in a non-stick pan. Place the tofu strips in the pan and fry until lightly browned. Place tofu on a plate to cool.
5. Pour hot water into a large shallow bowl and dip a rice wrapper in hot water. Once the wrapper is slightly soft, place it on a large plate and place two halves of the lettuce in the center of the wrapper.
6. Sprinkle two to three tablespoons of carrots and one to two tablespoons of sliced onion on top of the lettuce. Place one cooled tofu strip on top of vegetables.
7. Fold the sides in, and then fold the bottom up and roll tightly.
8. Refrigerate and serve cold.

Nutrition:

Calories: 156, Carbs: 20 g, Phosphorus: 93 mg, Potassium: 302 mg, Protein: 8 g, Sodium: 161 mg

Dessert Recipes

206. Baked Figs with Honey
Preparation Time: 10 minutes
Cooking Time: 15 minutes
Servings: 4
Ingredients:

- 4 figs

- 4 teaspoons honey
- 1 oz. Blue cheese, chopped

Directions:

1. Make the cross cuts in the figs and fill them with chopped Blue cheese.
2. Then sprinkle the figs with honey and wrap them in the foil.
3. Bake the figs for 15 minutes at 355°F.
4. Remove the figs from the foil and transfer them to the serving plates.

Nutrition:
Calories: 94, Fat: 2.2 g, Fiber: 1.9 g, Carbs: 18.1 g, Protein: 2.2 g

207. Cream Strawberry Pies
Preparation Time: 20 minutes
Cooking Time: 15 minutes
Servings: 6
Ingredients:

- 1 cup strawberries
- 7 oz. puff pastry
- 3 teaspoons butter, softened
- 3 teaspoons Erythritol
- ¼ teaspoon ground nutmeg
- 4 teaspoons cream

Directions:

1. Roll up the puff pastry and cut it into 6 squares.
2. Slice the strawberries.
3. Grease every puff pastry square with butter and then place the sliced strawberries on it.
4. Sprinkle every strawberry square with cream, ground nutmeg, and Erythritol.
5. Secure the edges of every puff pastry square in the shape of a pie.
6. Line the baking tray with baking paper.
7. Transfer the pies to the tray and place the tray in the oven.

8. Bake the pies for 15 minutes at 375°F.

Nutrition:
Calories: 209, Fat: 14.8 g, Fiber: 1 g, Carbs: 19.4 g, Protein: 2.6 g
208. Banana Muffins
Preparation Time: 10 minutes
Cooking Time: 12 minutes
Servings: 4
Ingredients:

- 4 tablespoons wheat flour
- 2 bananas, peeled
- 1 tablespoon Plain yogurt
- ½ teaspoon baking powder
- ¼ teaspoon lemon juice
- 1 teaspoon vanilla extract

Directions:

1. Mash the bananas with the help of the fork.
2. Then combine mashed bananas with flour, yogurt, baking powder, and lemon juice.
3. Add vanilla extract and stir the batter until smooth.
4. Fill ½ part of every muffin mold with banana batter and bake them for 12 minutes at 365°F.
5. Chill the muffins and remove them from the muffin molds.

Nutrition:
Calories: 87, Fat: 0.3 g, Fiber: 1.8 g, Carbs: 20.2 g, Protein: 1.7 g
209. Grilled Pineapple
Preparation Time: 7 minutes
Cooking Time: 5 minutes
Servings: 4
Ingredients:

- 10 oz. fresh pineapple
- ½ teaspoon ground ginger
- 1 tablespoon almond butter, softened

Directions:

1. Slice the pineapple into the Servings: pieces and brush with almond butter.
2. After this, sprinkle every pineapple piece with ground ginger.
3. Preheat the grill to 400°F.
4. Grill the pineapple for 2 minutes from each side.
5. The cooked fruit should have a light brown surface on both sides.

Nutrition:
Calories: 61, Fat: 2.4 g, Fiber: 1.4 g, Carbs: 10.2 g, Protein: 1.3 g

210. Coconut-Minutest Bars
Preparation Time: 35 minutes
Cooking Time: 1 minutes
Servings: 6
Ingredients:

- 3 tablespoons coconut butter
- ½ cup coconut flakes
- 1 egg, beaten
- 1 tablespoon cocoa powder
- 3 oz. graham crackers, crushed
- 2 tablespoons Erythritol
- 3 tablespoons butter
- 1 teaspoon minutest extract
- 1 teaspoon stevia powder
- 1 teaspoon of cocoa powder
- 1 tablespoon almond butter, melted

Directions:

1. Churn together coconut butter, coconut flakes, and 1 tablespoon of cocoa powder.
2. Then microwave the mixture for 1 minute or until it is melted.
3. Chill the liquid for 1 minute and fast add egg. Whisk it until homogenous and smooth.
4. Stir the liquid in the graham crackers and transfer it into the mold. Flatten it well with the help of the spoon.

5. After this, blend Erythritol, butter, minutest extract, and stevia powder.
6. When the mixture is fluffy, place it over the graham crackers layer.
7. Then mix up together 1 teaspoon of cocoa powder and almond butter.
8. Sprinkle the cooked mixture with cocoa liquid and flatten it.
9. Refrigerate the dessert for 30 minutes.
10. Then cut it into the bars.

Nutrition:
Calories: 213, Fat: 16.3 g, Fiber: 2.9 g, Carbs: 20 g, Protein: 3.5 g

211. Hummingbird Cake
Preparation Time: 20 minutes
Cooking Time: 30 minutes
Servings: 10
Ingredients:

- 1 cup of rice flour
- 1 cup coconut flour
- ½ cup wheat flour
- ½ cup Erythritol
- ½ teaspoon baking powder
- ¾ teaspoon salt
- ⅓ teaspoon ground cinnamon
- ½ cup olive oil
- 2 eggs, beaten
- 3 oz. pineapple, chopped
- 1 banana, chopped
- 3 tablespoons walnuts, chopped
- 6 tablespoons cream cheese

Directions:

1. In the mixing bowl combine the first 9 ingredients from the list above.
2. When the mixture is smooth and add the pineapple and bananas.
3. Add walnuts and mix up the dough well.

4. Put the dough into the baking pans and bake for 30 minutes at 355°F.
5. Then remove the cooked cakes from the oven and chill well.
6. Spread every cake with cream cheese and form them into 1 big cake.

Nutrition:
Calories: 278, Fat: 16 g, Fiber: 6 g, Carbs: 41.9 g, Protein: 5.5 g

212. Cool Mango Mousse
Preparation Time: 8 minutes
Cooking Time: 30 minutes
Servings: 6
Ingredients:

- 2 cups coconut cream, chipped
- 6 teaspoons honey
- 2 mangoes, chopped

Directions:

1. Blend honey and mango.
2. When the mixture is smooth, combine it with whipped cream and stir carefully.
3. Put the mango-cream mixture in the Servings: glasses and refrigerate for 30 minutes.

Nutrition:
Calories: 272, Fat: 19.5 g, Fiber: 3.6 g, Carbs: 27 g, Protein: 2.8 g

213. Sweet Potato Brownies
Preparation Time: 5 minutes
Cooking Time: 30 minutes
Servings: 6
Ingredients:

- 1 tablespoon cocoa powder
- 1 sweet potato, peeled, boiled
- ½ cup wheat flour
- 1 teaspoon baking powder
- 1 tablespoon butter

- 1 tablespoon olive oil
- 2 tablespoons Erythritol

Directions:

1. In the mixing bowl combine all ingredients.
2. Mix them well until you get a smooth batter.
3. After this, pour the brownie batter into the brownie mold and flatten it.
4. Bake it for 30 minutes at 365°F.
5. After this, cut the brownies into the serving bars.

Nutrition:
Calories: 95, Fat: 4.5 g, Fiber: 1.2 g, Carbs: 17.8 g, Protein: 1.6 g
214. Pumpkin Cookies
Preparation Time: 10 minutes
Cooking Time: 30 minutes
Servings: 6
Ingredients:

- 1 egg, beaten
- 1 teaspoon vanilla extract
- ½ teaspoon ground cinnamon
- 1 teaspoon ground turmeric
- 1 tablespoon butter, softened
- 1 cup wheat flour
- 1 teaspoon baking powder
- 4 tablespoons pumpkin puree
- 1 tablespoon Erythritol

Directions:

1. Put all ingredients in the mixing bowl and knead the soft and non-sticky dough.
2. After this, line the baking tray with baking paper.
3. Make 6 balls from the dough and press them gently with the help of the spoon.
4. Arrange the dough balls in the tray.
5. Bake the cookies for 30 minutes at 355°F.

6. Chill the cooked cookies well and store them in the glass jar.

Nutrition:
Calories: 111, Fat: 2.9 g, Fiber: 1.1 g, Carbs: 20.2 g, Protein: 3.2 g
215. Baked Plums
Preparation Time: 8 minutes
Cooking Time: 20 minutes
Servings: 4
Ingredients:

- 4 plums, pitted, halved, not soft
- 1 tablespoon peanuts, chopped
- 1 tablespoon honey
- ½ teaspoon lemon juice
- 1 teaspoon coconut oil

Directions:

1. Make the packet from the foil and place the plum halves in it.
2. Then sprinkle the plums with honey, lemon juice, coconut oil, and peanuts.
3. Bake the plums for 20 minutes at 350°F.

Nutrition:
Calories: 69, Fat: 2.5 g, Fiber: 1.1 g, Carbs: 12.7 g, Protein: 1.1 g
216. Apple Pie Bars
Preparation Time: 25 minutes
Cooking Time: 40 minutes
Servings: 18
Ingredients:
- 2 medium-sized apples
- ¾ cup of unsalted melted butter
- 1 cup of granulated sugar
- 1 cup of sour cream
- 1 teaspoon of vanilla extract
- 1 teaspoon of baking soda
- ½ teaspoon of salt (or exclude to reduce sodium)
- 2 cups of all-purpose flour
- ½ cup of brown sugar

- 1 teaspoon of cinnamon
- 2 tablespoons of milk
- 1 cup of powdered sugar

Directions:

1. Preheat oven to 350°F
2. Peel and chop the apples
3. Together, cream ½ cup of butter and granulated sugar in a bowl
4. Stir in the sour cream, baking soda, vanilla, salt, flour, and the chopped apples
5. Transfer the batter onto a 9 x 13-inch greased baking pan
6. Combine and mix two tablespoons of butter, brown sugar, and cinnamon in a small bowl, then sprinkle over the batter
7. Bake for about 35 to 40 minutes, then allow it cool completely
8. To make the icing, combine and mix two tablespoons of melted butter, powdered sugar, and milk, then drizzle over the top of the baked apple bar
9. Cut into 18 bars

Nutrition:

Calories: 246, Protein: 2 g, Carbs: 35 g, Fat: 11 g, Cholesterol: 26 mg, Sodium: 140 mg, Potassium: 72 mg, Phosphorus: 27 mg, Fiber: 0.6 g

217. Blueberry Peach Crisp

Preparation Time: 10 minutes

Cooking Time: 45 minutes

Servings: 10

Ingredients:

- 7 medium-sized fresh peaches
- 1 cup of blueberries
- ¼ cup of granulated sugar
- 1 tablespoon of lemon juice
- ¾ cup of all-purpose flour
- ¾ cup of packed brown sugar
- ½ cup of butter

Directions:

1. Preheat oven to 375°F
2. Pit and slice the peaches into ¾- inch slices

3. Use a cooking spray to spray a 12 x 9-inch baking dish, then place the peach slices and blueberries on top of the dish
4. Sprinkle over the fruit, sugar, and lemon juice
5. Use a small bowl to combine and mix the flour and brown sugar
6. Cut the butter into the flour mixture using two knives or pastry blender until it is crumbly. Sprinkle the crumbs on top of the fruit
7. Bake for about 45 minutes or until the fruit becomes soft and the crumbs are browned, then serve warm

Nutrition:
Calories: 238, Protein: 2 g, Carbs: 35 g, Fat: 10 g, Cholesterol: 24 mg, Sodium: 76 mg, Potassium: 240 mg, Phosphorus: 36 mg, Fiber: 2.1 g

218. Cherry Coffee Cake
Preparation Time: 10 minutes
Cooking Time: 40 minutes
Servings: 24
Ingredients:
- ½ cup of unsalted butter
- 2 eggs
- 1 cup of granulated sugar
- 1 cup of sour cream
- 1 teaspoon of vanilla
- 2 cups of all-purpose white flour
- 1 teaspoon of baking powder
- 1 teaspoon of baking soda
- 20 ounces of cherry pie filling

Directions:

1. Preheat the oven to 350°F
2. Set out the butter at room temperature to soften
3. Use a bowl to cream the butter, eggs, sour cream, sugar, and vanilla
4. Combine and mix the flour, baking powder, and baking soda in a separate bowl
5. Add the dry ingredients from step 4 to the creamed butter mixture. Mix properly, then pour the batter onto a greased 9 x 13-inch baking pan
6. Evenly spread the cherry pie filling over the batter

7. Bake for about 40 minutes or until it is golden brown

Nutrition:
Calories: 204, Protein: 3 g, Carbs: 30 g, Fat: 8 g, Cholesterol: 43 mg,
Sodium: 113 mg, Potassium: 72 mg, Phosphorus: 70 mg, Fiber: 0.5 g

219. Fruity Peach Crisp Dump
Preparation Time: 10 minutes
Cooking Time: 30 minutes
Servings: 12
Ingredients:
- 40 ounces of sliced canned peaches
- Non-stick cooking spray
- 15.25 ounces of boxed yellow dry mix cake
- ½ cup of unsalted margarine

Directions:

1. Preheat oven to 350°F
2. Spray the cooking spray over a 9 x 13-inch cake pan
3. Dump two cans of undrained peaches onto the cake pan, spreading evenly
4. Evenly sprinkle the yellow cake mix on top of the fruit, and dot with margarine
5. Bake for about 30 minutes

Nutrition:
Calories: 260, Protein: 1 g, Carbs: 44 g, Fat: 9 g, Sodium: 292 mg, Potassium: 107 mg, Phosphorus: 140 mg, Fiber: 0.7 g

220. Gingersnap Cookies
Preparation Time: 10 minutes
Cooking Time: 1hr 10 minutes
Servings: 24
Ingredients:
- 2 cups of all-purpose white flour
- 3 teaspoons of baking soda
- 1 teaspoon of ground cloves
- 1 teaspoon of ground ginger
- 1 teaspoon of ground cinnamon
- 1 stick of unsalted softened butter
- 1 cup of granulated sugar

- 1 egg
- 2 tablespoons of molasses

Directions:

1. Sift together, the flour, baking soda, ginger, cloves, and cinnamon
2. Cream the butter using a mixer until it becomes light and fluffy, add sugar gradually, then blend in the egg and molasses
3. Pour in a little amount of the flour mixture at a time until a dough is formed
4. Cover and store in the refrigerator for 1 hour or overnight
5. Preheat oven to 350°F
6. Form the dough into a heaped teaspoon ball size, and place 2-inch apart on top of a greased cookie sheet. Slightly flatten each ball
7. Bake for about 8 to 10 minutes, then cool on a wire rack
8. Make four dozen cookies

Nutrition:
Calories: 108, Protein: 1 g, Carbs: 17 g, Fat: 4 g, Cholesterol: 20 mg, Sodium: 162 mg, Potassium: 40 mg, Phosphorus: 14 mg, Fiber: 0.3 g

221. Lemon Icebox Pie
Preparation Time: 4hr 10 minutes
Cooking Time: 0 minutes
Servings: 8
Ingredients:
- ½ cup of water
- 1 small packet of Knox unflavored gelatin
- 8 ounces of light sour cream
- 2½ cups of fat-free Reddi-Wip dairy whipped topping
- ¼ cup of lemon juice
- ⅓ cup of granulated sugar
- ¼ teaspoon of lemon extract
- 6 drops of yellow food coloring
- 1 graham (9-inch) cracker pie crust

Directions:

1. Dissolve the gelatin into ½ cup of boiling water, and allow it to stand for about five minutes

2. Combine and mix the sour cream, 2 cups of whipped topping, lemon juice, sugar, lemon extract, and food coloring. Stir in the dissolved gelatin

3. Pour the mixture into a pie shell, and store in the refrigerator for about 4 hours or until it is set

4. Cut into slices, topping each with one tablespoon of the remaining whipped topping

Nutrition:
Calories: 253, Protein: 4 g, Carbs: 35 g, Fat: 11 g, Cholesterol: 13 mg, Sodium: 210 mg, Potassium: 116 mg, Phosphorus: 54 mg, Fiber: 0.5 g

222. Strawberry Pavlova
Preparation Time: 30 minutes
Cooking Time: 1hr 15 minutes
Servings: 8
Ingredients:
- 6 large egg white
- ⅛ teaspoon of salt (or exclude to reduce sodium)
- 2 cups and two tablespoons of granulated sugar
- 1½ teaspoons of vinegar
- 2½ teaspoons of vanilla extract
- 8 ounces of heavy whipping cream
- 4 cups of fresh sliced strawberries

Directions:

1. Preheat oven to 300°F.

2. Set out the egg white at room temperature, slice the strawberries, and keep aside

3. Beat the egg white with salt until soft peaks are formed. Add 2 cups of sugar, one tablespoon at a time, and beat properly after each addition. Fold in the vinegar gently, adding 1½ teaspoons of vanilla

4. Use an 8-inch round, and ungreased cookie sheet to smooth in the mixture

5. Bake for about 45 minutes, then allow the shell to set for about 1 hour with the oven door closed. Remove from the oven, allowing it to cool completely

6. Add sugar, whipping cream, and the remaining 1 teaspoon of vanilla into a bowl, whipping with a mixer until it becomes

stiff. Place the whipped cream in the freezer for about 10-15 minutes

7. Fill the top of the Pavlova shell from step 5 with the whipped topping and sliced berries

Nutrition:
Calories: 355, Protein: 4g, Carbs: 60 g, Fat: 11 g, Cholesterol: 39 mg, Sodium: 90 mg, Potassium: 175 mg, Phosphorus: 39 mg, Fiber: 1.0 g

223. Snickerdoodles
Preparation Time: 15 minutes
Cooking Time: 10 minutes
Servings: 24
Ingredients:

- 2¾ cups of all-purpose white flour
- 1¾ cups of sugar (divided use)
- 1 cup of softened butter
- 2 eggs
- 2 teaspoons cream of tartar
- 1 teaspoon of baking soda
- 1 teaspoon of vanilla
- 1½ teaspoon of ground cinnamon

Directions:

1. Preheat oven to 400°F
2. Use a large bowl to combine and mix all the cookie ingredients, excluding the cinnamon and leaving out ¼ of the sugar
3. Using a small bowl, stir in the remaining sugar and the cinnamon
4. Form 1-inch of balls and roll into the sugar mixture
5. Use an ungreased cookie sheet to place in the dough balls, 2-inch apart
6. Bake for about 8 to 10 minutes or until it is browned

Nutrition:
Calories: 185, Protein: 2 g, Carbs: 24 g, Fat: 9 g, Cholesterol: 39 mg, Sodium: 60 mg, Potassium: 66 mg, Phosphorus: 26 mg, Fiber: 0.5 g

224. Bread Pudding
Preparation Time: 15 minutes
Cooking Time: 40 minutes

Servings: 6
Ingredients:
- 2 large eggs
- 2 egg white
- 1½ cups of almond milk
- 2 tablespoons of honey
- 1 teaspoon of vanilla
- 2 tablespoons rum or 1 teaspoon rum extract
- 4 slices of raisin bread

Directions:

1. Preheat oven to 325°F
2. Use a non-stick cooking spray to spray an 8-inch round baking dish
3. Beat the eggs and egg white in a large mixing bowl until it is foamy. Beat in the almond milk, vanilla, honey, and the rum or rum extract
4. Cut the bread into cubes, stir into the egg mixture then spread over the baking dish
5. Bake for about 35 to 40 minutes or until it comes out clean when a knife is inserted at the center
6. Spoon out warm pudding into dishes to serve

Nutrition:
Calories: 124, Protein: 5 g, Carbs: 19 g, Fat: 3 g, Cholesterol: 62 mg, Sodium: 148 mg, Potassium: 115 mg, Phosphorus: 59 mg, Fiber: 1.0 g

225. Frozen Fruit Delight
Preparation Time: 3hr
Cooking Time: 0 minutes
Servings: 10
Ingredients:
- ⅓ cup of maraschino cherries
- 8 ounces of canned crushed pineapple
- 8 ounces of reduced-fat sour cream
- 1 tablespoon of lemon juice
- 1 cup of sliced strawberries
- ½ cup of sugar
- ⅛ teaspoon of salt
- 3 cups of Reddi-Wip dairy whipped topping

Directions:

1. Chop the cherries and drain the pineapple
2. Place all the ingredients into a medium-sized bowl except the whipped topping. Mix until well blended, then fold in the whipped topping.
3. Place the mixture into a freezable plastic container. Freeze for about 2 to 3 hours or until it is hardened

Nutrition:
Calories: 133, Protein: 1 g, Carbs: 21 g, Fat: 5 g, Cholesterol: 21 mg, Sodium: 5 9mg, Potassium: 99 mg, Phosphorus: 36 mg, Calcium: 47 mg, Fiber: 0.8 g

226. Tart Apple Granita
Preparation Time: 15 minutes, plus 4 hours freezing time
Cooking Time: 0 minutes
Servings: 4
Instructions:
- ½ cup granulated sugar
- ½ cup water
- 2 cups unsweetened apple juice
- ¼ cup freshly squeezed lemon juice

Directions:

1. In a small saucepan over medium-high heat, heat the sugar and water.
2. Bring the mixture to a boil and then reduce the heat to low and simmer for about 15 minutes or until the liquid has reduced by half.
3. Remove the pan from the heat and pour the liquid into a large shallow metal pan.
4. Let the liquid cool for about 30 minutes and then stir in the apple juice and lemon juice.
5. Place the pan in the freezer.
6. After 1 hour, run a fork through the liquid to break up any ice crystals that have formed. Scrape down the sides as well.
7. Place the pan back in the freezer and repeat the stirring and scraping every 20 minutes, creating slush.

8. Serve when the mixture is completely frozen and looks like crushed ice, after about 3 hours.

Nutrition:
Calories: 157, Phosphorus: 10 mg, Potassium: 141 mg, Sodium: 5 mg

227. Lemon-Lime Sherbet
Preparation Time: 5 minutes, plus 3 hours chilling time
Cooking Time: 15 minutes
Servings: 8
Ingredients:
- 2 cups of water
- 1 cup granulated sugar
- 3 tablespoons lemon zest, divided
- ½ cup freshly squeezed lemon juice
- Zest of 1 lime
- Juice of 1 lime
- ½ cup heavy (whipping) cream

Directions:

1. Place a large saucepan over medium-high heat and add the water, sugar, and 2 tablespoons of the lemon zest.
2. Bring the mixture to a boil and then reduce the heat and simmer for 15 minutes.
3. Transfer the mixture to a large bowl and add the remaining 1 tablespoon lemon zest, the lemon juice, lime zest, and lime juice.
4. Chill the mixture in the fridge until completely cold, about 3 hours.
5. Whisk in the heavy cream and transfer the mixture to an ice cream maker.
6. Freeze according to the manufacturer's instructions.

Nutrition:
Calories: 151, Fat: 6 g, Carbs: 26 g, Phosphorus: 10 mg, Potassium: 27 mg, Sodium: 6 mg

228. Tropical Vanilla Snow Cone
Preparation Time: 15 minutes, plus freezing time
Cooking Time: 0 minutes
Servings: 4

Ingredients:
- 1 cup canned peaches
- 1 cup pineapple
- 1 cup of frozen strawberries
- 6 tablespoons water
- 2 tablespoons granulated sugar
- 1 tablespoon vanilla extract

Directions:

1. In a large saucepan, mix the peaches, pineapple, strawberries, water, and sugar over medium-high heat and bring to a boil.
2. Reduce the heat to low and simmer the mixture, stirring occasionally, for 15 minutes.
3. Remove from the heat and let the mixture cool completely, for about 1 hour.
4. Stir in the vanilla and transfer the fruit mixture to a food processor or blender.
5. Purée until smooth and pour the purée into a 9-by-13-inch glass baking dish.
6. Cover and place the dish in the freezer overnight.
7. When the fruit mixture is completely frozen, use a fork to scrape the sorbet until you have flaked flavored ice.
8. Scoop the ice flakes into 4 serving dishes.

Nutrition:
Calories: 92, Carbs: 22 g, Phosphorus: 17 mg, Potassium: 145 mg, Sodium: 4 mg, Protein: 1 g

229. Pavlova with Peaches
Preparation Time: 30 minutes
Cooking Time: 1 hour, plus cooling time
Servings: 8
Ingredients:
- 4 large egg whites, at room temperature
- ½ teaspoon cream of tartar
- 1 cup superfine sugar
- ½ teaspoon pure vanilla extract
- 2 cups drained canned peaches in juice

Directions:

1. Preheat the oven to 225°F.
2. Line a baking sheet with parchment paper, set aside.
3. In a large bowl, beat the egg whites for about 1 minute or until soft peaks form.
4. Beat in the cream of tartar.
5. Add the sugar, 1 tablespoon at a time, until the egg whites are very stiff and glossy. Do not overbeat.
6. Beat in the vanilla.
7. Evenly spoon the meringue onto the baking sheet so that you have 8 rounds.
8. Use the back of the spoon to create an indentation in the middle of each round.
9. Bake the meringues for about 1 hour or until a light brown crust forms.
10. Turn off the oven and let the meringues stand, still in the oven, overnight.
11. Remove the meringues from the sheet and place them on Servings: plates.
12. Spoon the peaches, dividing evenly, into the centers of the meringues, and serve.
13. Store any unused meringues in a sealed container at room temperature for up to 1 week.

Nutrition:
Calories: 132, Carbs: 32 g, Phosphorus: 7 mg, Potassium: 95 mg, Sodium: 30 mg, Protein: 2 g

230. Baked Peaches with Cream Cheese
Preparation Time: 10 minutes
Cooking Time: 15 minutes
Servings: 4
Ingredients:

- 1 cup plain cream cheese, at room temperature
- ½ cup crushed Meringue Cookies (here)
- ¼ teaspoon ground cinnamon
- Pinch ground nutmeg
- 8 canned peach halves, in juice
- 2 tablespoons honey

Directions:

1. Preheat the oven to 350°F.
2. Line a baking sheet with parchment paper, set aside.
3. In a small bowl, stir together the cream cheese, meringue cookies, cinnamon, and nutmeg.
4. Spoon the cream cheese mixture evenly into the cavities in the peach halves.
5. Place the peaches on the baking sheet and bake for about 15 minutes or until the fruit is soft and the cheese is melted.
6. Remove the peaches from the baking sheet onto plates, 2 per person, and drizzle with honey before serving.

Nutrition:
Calories: 260, Fat: 20 g, Carbs: 19 g, Phosphorus: 74 mg, Potassium: 198 mg, Sodium: 216 mg, Protein: 4 g

231. Sweet Cinnamon Custard
Preparation Time: 20 minutes, plus 1-hour chilling time
Cooking Time: 1 hour
Servings: 6
Ingredients:

- Unsalted butter, for greasing the ramekins
- 1½ cups plain rice milk
- 4 eggs
- ¼ cup granulated sugar
- 1 teaspoon pure vanilla extract
- ½ teaspoon ground cinnamon
- Cinnamon sticks, for garnish (optional)

Directions:

1. Preheat the oven to 325°F.
2. Lightly grease 6 (4-ounce) ramekins and place them in a baking dish, set aside.
3. In a large bowl, whisk together the rice milk, eggs, sugar, vanilla, and cinnamon until the mixture is very smooth.
4. Pour the mixture through a fine sieve into a pitcher.
5. Evenly divide the custard mixture among the ramekins.

6. Fill the baking dish with hot water, taking care not to get any water in the ramekins, until the water reaches halfway up the sides of the ramekins.
7. Bake for about 1 hour or until the custards are set and a knife inserted in the center of one of the custards comes out clean.
8. Remove the custards from the oven and take the ramekins out of the water.
9. Cool on wire racks for 1 hour and then transfer the custards to the refrigerator to chill for an additional hour.
10. Garnish each custard with a cinnamon stick, if desired.

Nutrition:
Calories: 110, Fat: 4 g, Carbs: 14 g, Phosphorus: 100 mg, Potassium: 64 mg, Sodium: 71 mg, Protein: 4 g

232. Raspberry Brûlée
Preparation Time: 15 minutes
Cooking Time: 1 minute
Servings: 4
Ingredients:

- ½ cup light sour cream
- ½ cup plain cream cheese, at room temperature
- ¼ cup brown sugar, divided
- ¼ teaspoon ground cinnamon
- 1 cup fresh raspberries

Directions:

1. Preheat the oven to broil.
2. In a small bowl, beat together the sour cream, cream cheese, 2 tablespoons brown sugar, and cinnamon for about 4 minutes or until the mixture is very smooth and fluffy.
3. Evenly divide the raspberries among 4 (4-ounce) ramekins.
4. Spoon the cream cheese mixture over the berries and smooth the tops.
5. Store the ramekins in the refrigerator, covered, until you are ready to serve the dessert.
6. Sprinkle ½ tablespoon brown sugar evenly over each ramekin.
7. Place the ramekins on a baking sheet and broil 4 inches from

the heating element until the sugar is caramelized and golden brown.

8. Remove from the oven. Let the brûlées sit for 1 minute then serve.

Nutrition:
Calories: 188, Fat: 13 g, Carbs: 16 g, Phosphorus: 60 mg, Potassium: 158 mg, Sodium: 132 mg, Protein: 3 g

233. Vanilla-Infused Couscous Pudding
Preparation Time: 20 minutes
Cooking Time: 20 minutes
Servings: 6
Ingredients:

- 1½ cups plain rice milk
- ½ cup water
- 1 vanilla bean, split
- ½ cup honey
- ¼ teaspoon ground cinnamon
- 1 cup couscous

Directions:

1. In a large saucepan, mix the rice milk, water, and vanilla bean over medium heat.
2. Bring the milk to a gentle simmer, reduce the heat to low, and let the milk simmer for 10 minutes to allow the vanilla flavor to infuse into the milk.
3. Remove the saucepan from the heat.
4. Take out the vanilla bean and, using the tip of a paring knife, scrape the seeds from the pod into the warm milk.
5. Stir in the honey and cinnamon.
6. Stir in the couscous, cover the pan, and let it stand for 10 minutes.
7. With a fork, fluff the couscous before serving.

Nutrition:
Calories: 334, Fat: 1 g, Carbs: 77 g, Phosphorus: 119 mg, Potassium: 118 mg, Sodium: 41 mg, Protein: 6 g

234. Honey Bread Pudding

Preparation Time: 15 minutes, plus 3 hours soaking time
Cooking Time: 40 minutes
Servings: 6
Ingredients:

- Unsalted butter, for greasing the baking dish
- 1½ cups plain rice milk
- 2 eggs
- 2 large egg whites
- ¼ cup honey
- 1 teaspoon pure vanilla extract
- 6 cups cubed white bread

Directions:

1. Lightly grease an 8-by-8-inch baking dish with butter, set aside.
2. In a medium bowl, whisk together the rice milk, eggs, egg whites, honey, and vanilla.
3. Add the bread cubes and stir until the bread is coated.
4. Transfer the mixture to the baking dish and cover with plastic wrap.
5. Store the dish in the refrigerator for at least 3 hours.
6. Preheat the oven to 325°F.
7. Remove the plastic wrap from the baking dish and bake the pudding for 35 to 40 minutes or until golden brown and a knife inserted in the center comes out clean.
8. Serve warm.

Nutrition:

Calories: 167, Fat: 3 g, Carbs: 30 g, Phosphorus: 95 mg, Potassium: 93 mg, Sodium: 189 mg, Protein: 6 g

235. Rhubarb Crumble

Preparation Time: 15 minutes
Cooking Time: 30 minutes
Servings: 6
Ingredients:

- Unsalted butter, for greasing the baking dish

- 1 cup all-purpose flour
- ½ cup brown sugar
- ½ teaspoon ground cinnamon
- ½ cup unsalted butter, at room temperature
- 1 cup chopped rhubarb
- 2 apples, peeled, cored, and sliced thin
- 2 tablespoons granulated sugar
- 2 tablespoons water

Directions:

1. Preheat the oven to 325°F.
2. Lightly grease an 8-by-8-inch baking dish with butter, set aside.
3. In a small bowl, stir together the flour, sugar, and cinnamon until well combined.
4. Add the butter and rub the mixture between your fingers until it resembles coarse crumbs.
5. In a medium saucepan, mix the rhubarb, apple, sugar, and water over medium heat and cook for about 20 minutes or until the rhubarb is soft.
6. Spoon the fruit mixture into the baking dish and evenly top with the crumble.
7. Bake the crumble for 20 to 30 minutes or until golden brown.
8. Serve hot.

Nutrition:
Calories: 450, Fat: 23 g, Carbs: 60 g, Phosphorus: 51 mg, Potassium: 181 mg, Sodium: 10 mg, Protein: 4 g

236. Buttery Pound Cake
Preparation Time: 20 minutes
Cooking Time: 75 minutes
Servings: 20
Ingredients:

- Unsalted butter, for greasing the baking pan
- All-purpose flour, for dusting the baking pan
- 2 cups of unsalted butter, at room temperature
- 3 cups of granulated sugar
- 6 eggs, at room temperature

- 1 tablespoon of pure vanilla extract
- 4 cups of all-purpose flour
- ¾ cup of unsweetened rice milk

Directions:

1. Preheat the oven to 325°F.
2. Grease your Bundt pan (10-inch) with butter and dust with flour, set aside.
3. Use a large bowl, make sure to beat the butter and sugar with a hand mixer for about 4 minutes or until very fluffy and pale.
4. Add the eggs, one at a time, beating well after each addition and scraping down the sides of the bowl.
5. Beat in the vanilla.
6. Add the flour and rice milk, alternating in 3 additions, with the flour first and last.
7. Spoon the batter into the Bundt pan.
8. Bake for 1 hour and 15 minutes or until the top of the cake is golden brown and the cake springs back when lightly pressed.
9. Cool the cake in the Bundt pan on a wire rack for 10 minutes.
10. Remove the cake from the pan to a wire rack and cool completely before serving.

Nutrition:
Calories: 389, Fat: 20 g, Carbs: 50 g, Phosphorus: 67 mg, Potassium: 57 mg, Sodium: 28 mg, Protein: 5 g

237. Pudding Glass with Banana and Whipped Cream
Preparation Time: 10 minutes
Cooking Time: 8 minutes
Servings: 2
Ingredients:

- 2 portions of banana cream pudding mix
- 2 ½ cups of rice milk
- 8 oz. of dairy whipped cream
- 12 oz. of vanilla wafers

Directions:

1. Put vanilla wafers in a pan, and in another bowl, mix banana cream pudding and rice milk.
2. Boil the ingredients, blending them slowly.
3. Pour the mixture over the wafers and make 2 or 3 layers.
4. Put the pan in the fridge for one hour and afterward spread the whipped topping over the dessert.
5. Put it back in the fridge for 2 hours and serve it cool in transparent glasses. Serve and enjoy!

Nutrition:
Calories: 255, Protein: 3 g, Sodium: 275 mg, Potassium: 50 mg, Phosphorus: 40 mg

238. Chocolate Beet Cake
Preparation Time: 10 minutes
Cooking Time: 50 minutes
Servings: 12
Ingredients:

- 3 cups of grated beets
- ¼ cup of canola oil
- 4 eggs
- 4 oz. of unsweetened chocolate
- 2 tsp. of Phosphorus-free baking powder
- 2 cups of all-purpose flour
- 1 cup of sugar

Directions:

1. Set your oven to 325°F. Grease two 8-inch cake pans.
2. Mix the baking powder, flour, and sugar. Set aside.
3. Chop up the chocolate as finely as you can and melt using a double boiler. A microwave can also be used, but don't let it burn.
4. Allow it to cool and then mix in the oil and eggs.
5. Mix all the wet ingredients into the flour mixture and combine everything until well mixed.
6. Fold the beets in and pour the batter into the cake pans.
7. Let them bake for 40 to 50 minutes. To know it's done, the toothpick should come out clean when inserted into the cake.

8. Remove from the oven and allow them to cool.
9. Once cool, invert over a plate to remove.
10. This is great when served with whipped cream and fresh berries. Enjoy!

Nutrition:
Calories: 270, Protein: 6 g, Sodium: 109 mg, Potassium: 299 mg, Phosphorus: 111 mg

239. Strawberry Pie
Preparation Time: 25 minutes
Cooking Time: 3 hours
Servings: 8
Ingredients:
For the Crust:

- 1 ½ cups of Graham cracker crumbs
- 5 tbsp. of unsalted butter, at room temperature
- 2 tbsp. of sugar

For the Pie:

- 1 ½ tsp. of gelatin powder
- 3 tbsp. of cornstarch
- ¾ cup of sugar
- 5 cups of sliced strawberries, divided
- 1 cup of water

Directions:
For the crust:

1. Heat your oven to 375°F. Grease a pie pan.
2. Combine the butter, crumbs, and sugar, and then press them into your pie pan.
3. Bake the crust for 10 to 15 minutes, until lightly browned.
4. Take out of the oven and let it cool completely.

For the pie:

1. Crush up a cup of strawberries.

2. Using a small pot, combine the sugar, water, gelatin, and cornstarch.
3. Bring the mixture in the pot up to a boil, lower the heat, and simmer until it has thickened.
4. Add in the crushed strawberries in the pot and let it simmer for another 5 minutes until the sauce has thickened up again.
5. Set it off the heat and pour it into a bowl.
6. Cool until it comes to room temperature.
7. Toss the remaining berries with the sauce so that it is well distributed and pour into the pie crust and spread it out into an even layer.
8. Refrigerate the pie until cold. This will take about 3 hours. Serve and enjoy!

Nutrition:
Calories: 265, Protein: 3 g, Sodium: 143 mg, Potassium: 183 mg, Phosphorus: 44 mg

240. Grape Skillet Galette
Preparation Time: 20 minutes
Cooking Time: 2 hours
Servings: 6
Ingredients:
For the Crust:

- ½ cup of unsweetened rice milk
- 4 tbsp. of cold butter
- 1 tbsp. of sugar
- 1 cup of all-purpose flour

For the Galette:

- 1 tbsp. of cornstarch
- ⅓ cup of sugar
- 1 egg white
- 2 cups of halved seedless grapes

Directions:
For the crust:

1. Add the sugar and the flour to a food processor and mix for a few seconds.
2. Place in the butter and pulse until it looks like a coarse meal.
3. Add in the rice milk and combine until the dough forms.
4. Place the dough on a clean surface and shape it into a disc.
5. Wrap it with plastic wrap and place it in the fridge for 2 hours.

For the galette:

1. Set your oven to 425°F.
2. Mix the cornstarch and sugar and toss the grapes in.
3. Unwrap the dough and roll out on a floured surface.
4. Press it into a 14-inch circle and place it in a cast-iron skillet.
5. Add the grape filling in the center and spread out to fill, leaving a 2-inch crust. Fold the edge over.
6. Brush the crust with egg white and cook for 20 to 25 minutes. The crust should be golden.
7. Allow to rest for 20 minutes before you serve. Enjoy!

Nutrition:
Calories: 172, Protein: 2 g, Sodium: 65 mg, Potassium: 69 mg, Phosphorus: 21 mg

241. Pumpkin Cheesecake
Preparation Time: 20 minutes
Cooking Time: 50 minutes
Servings: 2
Ingredients:

- 1 egg white
- 1 wafer crumb, 9-inch pie crust
- ½ small bowl of granular sugar
- 1 tsp. of vanilla extract
- 1 tsp. of pumpkin pie flavoring
- ½ bowl of pumpkin cream
- ½ small bowl of liquid egg substitute
- 8 tbsp. of frozen topping, for desserts
- 16 oz. of cream cheese

Directions:

1. Brush pie crust with egg white and cook for 5 minutes in a Preheated oven from 375°F from 375°F now down to 350°F.
2. In a large cup, put together sugar, vanilla, and cream cheese, beating with a mixer until smooth.
3. Beat the egg substitute and add pumpkin cream with pie flavoring: blend everything until softened.
4. Put the pumpkin mixture in a pie shell and bake for 50 minutes to set the center.
5. Then let the pie cool down and then put it in the fridge. When you wish to, serve it in 8 slices, putting some topping on it. Serve and enjoy!

Nutrition:
Calories: 364, Protein: 5 g, Sodium: 245 mg, Potassium: 125 mg, Phosphorus: 65 mg

242. Small Chocolate Cakes
Preparation Time: 5 minutes
Cooking Time: 15 minutes
Servings: 2
Ingredients:

- 1 box of angel food cake mix
- 1 box of lemon cake mix
- Water
- Non-stick cooking spray or batter
- Dark chocolate small, squared chops and chocolate powder

Directions:

1. Use a transparent kitchen cooking bag and put lemon cake mix, angel food mix, and chocolate chips inside.
2. Mix everything and add water to prepare a small cupcake.
3. Put the mix in a mold to prepare a cupcake containing the ingredients and put it in the microwave for a minute at a high temperature.
4. Slip the cupcake out of the mold and put it on a dish, let it cool, and put some more chocolate crumbs on it. Serve and enjoy!

Nutrition:

Calories: 95, Protein: 1 g, Sodium: 162 mg, Potassium: 15 mg, Phosphorus: 80 mg

243. Strawberry Whipped Cream Cake
Preparation Time: 10 minutes
Cooking Time: 20 minutes
Servings: 2
Ingredients:

- 1 pint of whipping cream
- 2 tbsp. of gelatin
- ½ glass of cold water
- 1 glass of boiling water
- 3 tbsp. of lemon juice
- 1 orange glass juice
- 1 tsp. of sugar
- ¾ cup of sliced strawberries
- 1 large angel food cake or light sponge cake

Directions:

1. Put the gelatin in cold water, then add hot water and blend. Add orange and lemon juice, also add some sugar and go on blending.
2. Refrigerate and leave it there until you see it is starting to gel.
3. Whip half portion of cream and add it to the mixture along with strawberries, put wax paper in the bowl, and cut the cake into small pieces.
4. In between the pieces, add the whipped cream and put everything in the fridge for one night.
5. When you take out the cake, add some whipped cream on top and decorate with some more fruit. Serve and enjoy!

Nutrition:
Calories: 355, Protein: 4 g, Sodium: 275 mg, Potassium: 145 mg, Phosphorus: 145 mg

244. Sweet Cracker Pie Crust
Preparation Time: 5 minutes
Cooking Time: 10 minutes
Servings: 2

Ingredients:

- 1 bowl of gelatin cracker crumbs
- ¼ small cup of sugar
- Unsalted butter

Directions:

1. Mix sweet cracker crumbs, butter, and sugar.
2. Put in the over Preheat at 375°F.
3. Bake for 7 minutes, putting it in a greased pie.
4. Let the pie cool before adding any kind of filling. Serve and enjoy!

Nutrition:
Calories: 205, Protein: 2 g, Sodium: 208 mg, Potassium: 67 mg, Phosphorus: 22 mg

245. Old-Fashioned Apple Kuchen
Preparation Time: 25 minutes
Cooking Time: 60 minutes
Servings: 16
Ingredients:

- Unsalted butter, for greasing the baking sheet
- 1 cup of unsalted butter, at room temperature
- 2 cups of granulated sugar
- 2 eggs, beaten
- 2 teaspoons of pure vanilla extract
- 2 cups of all-purpose flour
- 1 teaspoon of Ener-G baking soda substitute
- 2 teaspoons of ground cinnamon
- ½ teaspoon of ground nutmeg
- Pinch ground allspice
- 2 large apples (about 3 cups) peeled, cored, and diced

Directions:

1. Preheat the oven to 350°F.
2. Grease a 9-by-13-inch glass baking sheet, set aside.

3. Cream together the butter and sugar with a hand mixer until light and fluffy, for about 3 minutes.
4. Add the eggs and vanilla and beat until combined, scraping down the sides of the bowl, about 1 minute.
5. Stir the flour, baking soda substitute, cinnamon, nutmeg, and allspice all together using a large bowl.
6. Add all the dry ingredients to your wet ingredients, then stir to combine everything.
7. Stir in the apple and spoon the batter into the baking sheet.
8. Bake for about 1 hour or until the cake is golden.
9. Cool the cake on a wire rack.
10. Serve warm or chilled.

Nutrition:
Calories: 368, Fat: 16 g, Carbs: 53 g, Phosphorus: 46 mg, Potassium: 68 mg, Sodium: 15 mg, Protein: 3 g

Smoothies and Juices

246. Almonds & Blueberries Smoothie
Preparation Time: 5 minutes
Cooking Time: 0 minutes
Servings: 2
Ingredients:

- ¼ cup ground almonds, unsalted
- 1 cup fresh blueberries
- Fresh juice of a 1 lemon
- 1 cup fresh Kale leaves
- ½ cup coconut water
- 1 cup water
- 2 Tbsp. plain yogurt (optional)

Directions:

1. Dump all ingredients in your high-speed blender, and blend until your smoothie is smooth.
2. Pour the mixture into a chilled glass.
3. Serve and enjoy!

Nutrition:
Calories: 110, Carbs: 8 g, Protein: 2 g, Fat: 7 g, Fiber: 2 g

247.   **Almonds and Zucchini Smoothie**
Preparation Time: 5 minutes
Cooking Time: 0 minutes
Servings: 2
Ingredients:

- 1 cup zucchini, cooked and mashed - unsalted
- 1 ½ cups almond milk
- 1 Tbsp. almond butter (plain, unsalted)
- 1 tsp pure almond extract
- 2 Tbsp. ground almonds or Macadamia almonds
- ½ cup water
- 1 cup Ice cubes crushed (optional, for serving)

Directions:

1. Dump all ingredients from the list above in your fast-speed blender, blend for 45 - 60 seconds, or to taste.
2. Serve with crushed ice.

Nutrition:
Calories: 322, Carbs: 6 g, Protein: 6 g, Fat: 30 g, Fiber: 3.5 g

248.   **Avocado with Walnut Butter Smoothie**
Preparation Time: 5 minutes
Cooking Time: 0 minutes
Servings: 2
Ingredients:

- 1 avocado (diced)
- 1 cup baby spinach
- 1 cup coconut milk (canned)
- 1 Tbsp. walnut butter, unsalted
- 2 Tbsp. natural sweeteners such as Stevia, Erythritol, or Truvia

Directions:

1. Place all ingredients into a food processor or a blender, blend until smooth or to taste.
2. Add walnut butter.
3. Drink and enjoy!

Nutrition:
Calories: 364, Carbs: 7 g, Protein: 8 g, Fat: 35 g, Fiber: 5.5 g
249.   **Baby Spinach and Dill Smoothie**
Preparation Time: 5 minutes
Cooking Time: 0 minutes
Servings: 2
Ingredients:

- 1 cup of fresh baby spinach leaves
- 2 tbsp. of fresh dill, chopped
- 1 ½ cup of water
- ½ avocado, chopped into cubes
- 1 tbsp. chia seeds (optional)
- 2 tbsp. of natural sweetener Stevia or Erythritol (optional)

Directions:

1. Place all ingredients into a fast-speed blender. Beat until smooth and all Ingredients united well.
2. Serve and enjoy!

Nutrition:
Calories: 136, Carbs: 8 g, Protein: 7 g, Fat: 10 g, Fiber: 9 g
250.   **Blueberries and Coconut Smoothie**
Preparation Time: 5 minutes
Cooking Time: 0 minutes
Servings: 5
Ingredients:

- 1 cup of frozen blueberries, unsweetened
- 1 cup Stevia or Erythritol sweetener
- 2 cups of coconut milk (canned)
- 1 cup of fresh spinach leaves
- 2 tbsp. shredded coconut (unsweetened)

- ¾ cup water

Directions:

1. Place all ingredients from the list in the food processor or your strong blender.
2. Blend for 45 - 60 seconds or to taste.
3. Ready for a drink! Serve!

Nutrition:
Calories: 190, Carbs: 8 g, Protein: 3 g, Fat: 18 g, Fiber: 2 g
251. **Collard Greens and Cucumber Smoothie**
Preparation Time: 15 minutes
Cooking Time: 0 minutes
Servings: 2
Ingredients:

- 1 cup Collard greens
- A few fresh peppermints leaves
- 1 big cucumber
- 1 lime, freshly juiced
- ½ cups avocado sliced
- 1 ½ cup water
- 1 cup crushed ice
- ¼ cup of natural sweetener Erythritol or Stevia (optional)

Directions:

1. Rinse and clean your Collard greens from any dirt.
2. Place all ingredients in a food processor or blender,
3. Blend until all ingredients in your smoothie is combined well.
4. Pour in a glass and drink. Enjoy!

Nutrition:
Calories: 123, Carbs: 8 g, Protein: 4 g, Fat: 11 g, Fiber: 6 g
252. **Creamy Dandelion Greens and Celery Smoothie**
Preparation Time: 10 minutes
Cooking Time: 0 minutes

Servings: 2
Ingredients:

- 1 handful of raw dandelion greens
- 2 celery sticks
- 2 tbsp. chia seeds
- 1 small piece of ginger, minced
- ½ cup almond milk
- ½ cup of water
- ½ cup plain yogurt

Directions:

1. Rinse and clean dandelion leaves from any dirt, add in a high-speed blender.
2. Clean the ginger, keep only the inner part, and cut into small slices, add in a blender.
3. Add all remaining ingredients and blend until smooth.
4. Serve and enjoy!

Nutrition:
Calories: 58, Carbs: 5 g, Protein: 3 g, Fat: 6 g, Fiber: 3 g

253.   Dark Turnip Greens Smoothie
Preparation Time: 10 minutes
Cooking Time: 0 minutes
Servings: 2
Ingredients:

- 1 cup of raw turnip greens
- 1 ½ cup of almond milk
- 1 tbsp. of almond butter
- ½ cup of water
- ½ tsp of cocoa powder, unsweetened
- 1 tbsp. of dark chocolate chips
- ¼ tsp of cinnamon
- A pinch of salt
- ½ cup of crushed ice

Directions:

1. Rinse and clean turnip greens from any dirt.
2. Place the turnip greens in your blender along with all other ingredients.
3. Blend it for 45 - 60 seconds or until done, smooth and creamy.
4. Serve with or without crushed ice.

Nutrition:
Calories: 131, Carbs: 6 g, Protein: 4 g, Fat: 10 g, Fiber: 2.5 g

254.   **Butter Pecan and Coconut Smoothie**
Preparation Time: 5 minutes
Cooking Time: 0 minutes
Servings: 2
Ingredients:

- 1 cup coconut milk, canned
- 1 scoop Butter Pecan powdered creamer
- 2 cups fresh spinach leaves, chopped
- ½ banana frozen or fresh
- 2 tbsp. stevia granulated sweetener to taste
- ½ cup water
- 1 cup ice cubes crushed

Directions:

1. Place Ingredients from the list above in your high-speed blender.
2. Blend for 35 - 50 seconds or until all ingredients are combined well.
3. Add less or more crushed ice.
4. Drink and enjoy!

Nutrition:
Calories: 268, Carbs: 7 g, Protein: 6 g, Fat: 26 g, Fiber: 1.5 g

255.   **Fresh Cucumber, Kale, and Raspberry Smoothie**
Preparation Time: 10 minutes
Cooking Time: 0 minutes
Servings: 3
Ingredients:

- 1 ½ cups of cucumber, peeled
- ½ cup raw kale leaves
- 1 ½ cups fresh raspberries
- 1 cup of almond milk
- 1 cup of water
- Ice cubes crushed (optional)
- 2 tbsp. natural sweetener (Stevia, Erythritol...etc.)

Directions:

1. Place all ingredients from the list in a food processor or high-speed blender, blend for 35 - 40 seconds.
2. Serve into chilled glasses.
3. Add more natural sweeter if you like. Enjoy!

Nutrition:
Calories: 70, Carbs: 8 g, Protein: 3 g, Fat: 6 g, Fiber: 5 g
256. The Green Minty Smoothie
Preparation Time: 10 minutes
Cooking Time: 0 minutes
Servings: 1
Ingredients:

- 1 stalk celery
- 2 cups of water
- 2 oz. almonds
- 1 packet Stevia
- 2 minutest leaves

Directions:

1. Add listed ingredients to a blender
2. Blend until you have a smooth and creamy texture
3. Serve chilled and enjoy!

Nutrition:
Calories: 417, Fat: 43 g, Carbs: 10 g, Protein: 5.5 g
257. Mocha Milk Shake
Preparation Time: 10 minutes

Cooking Time: 0 minutes
Servings: 1
Ingredients:

- 1 cup whole milk
- 2 tablespoons cocoa powder
- 2 pack stevia
- 1 cup brewed coffee, chilled
- 1 tablespoon coconut oil

Directions:

1. Add listed ingredients to a blender
2. Blend until you have a smooth and creamy texture
3. Serve chilled and enjoy!

Nutrition:
Calories: 293, Fat: 23 g, Carbs: 19 g, Protein: 10 g

258. Gut Cleansing Smoothie
Preparation Time: 10 minutes
Cooking Time: 0 minutes
Servings: 1
Ingredients:

- 1 ½ tablespoons coconut oil, unrefined
- ½ cup plain full-fat yogurt
- 1 tablespoon chia seeds
- 1 Serving: aloe vera leaves
- ½ cup frozen blueberries, unsweetened
- 1 tablespoon hemp hearts
- 1 cup of water
- 1 scoop Pinnaclife prebiotic fiber

Directions:

1. Add listed ingredients to a blender
2. Blend until you have a smooth and creamy texture
3. Serve chilled and enjoy!

Nutrition:
Calories: 409, Fat: 33 g, Carbs: 8 g, Protein: 12 g
259. Cabbage and Chia Glass
Preparation Time: 10 minutes
Cooking Time: 0 minutes
Servings: 2
Ingredients:

- ⅓ cup cabbage
- 1 cup cold unsweetened almond milk
- 1 tablespoon chia seeds
- ½ cup cherries
- ½ cup lettuce

Directions:

1. Add coconut milk to your blender
2. Cut cabbage and add to your blender
3. Place chia seeds in a coffee grinder and chop to powder, brush the powder into a blender
4. Pit the cherries and add them to the blender
5. Wash and dry the lettuce and chop
6. Add to the mix
7. Cover and blend on low followed by medium
8. Taste the texture and serve chilled!

Nutrition:
Calories: 409, Fat: 33 g, Carbs: 8 g, Protein: 12 g
260. Blueberry and Kale Mix
Preparation Time: 10 minutes
Cooking Time: 0 minutes
Servings: 1
Ingredients:

- ½ cup low-fat Greek Yogurt
- 1 cup baby kale greens
- 1 pack stevia
- 1 tablespoon MCT oil
- ¼ cup blueberries

- 1 tablespoon pepitas
- 1 tablespoon flaxseed, ground
- 1 ½ cups of water

Directions:

1. Add listed ingredients to a blender
2. Blend until you have a smooth and creamy texture
3. Serve chilled and enjoy!

Nutrition:
Calories: 307, Fat: 24 g, Carbs: 14 g, Protein: 9 g
261. Rosemary and Lemon Garden Smoothie
Preparation Time: 10 minutes
Cooking Time: 0 minutes
Servings: 1
Ingredients:

- ½ cup low-fat Greek Yogurt
- 1 cup garden greens
- 1 pack stevia
- 1 tablespoon olive oil
- 1 stalk fresh rosemary
- 1 tablespoon lemon juice, fresh
- 1 tablespoon pepitas
- 1 tablespoon flaxseed, ground
- 1 ½ cups of water

Directions:

1. Add listed ingredients to a blender
2. Blend until you have a smooth and creamy texture
3. Serve chilled and enjoy!

Nutrition:
Calories: 312, Fat: 25 g, Carbs: 14 g, Protein: 9 g
262. Melon and Coconut Dish
Preparation Time: 10 minutes
Cooking Time: 0 minutes

Servings: 1
Ingredients:

- ¼ cup low-fat Greek yogurt
- 1 pack stevia
- 1 tablespoon coconut oil
- ½ cup melon, sliced
- 1 tablespoon coconut flakes, unsweetened
- 1 tablespoon chia seeds
- 1 and ½ cups of water

Directions:

1. Add listed ingredients to a blender
2. Blend until you have a smooth and creamy texture
3. Serve chilled and enjoy!

Nutrition:
Calories: 278, Fat: 21 g, Carbs: 15 g, Protein: 6 g
263. Strawberry Glass
Preparation Time: 10 minutes
Cooking Time: 0 minutes
Servings: 2
Ingredients:

- 1-2 handful baby greens
- 3 medium kale leaves
- 5-8 minutest leaves
- 1-inch piece ginger, peeled
- 1 avocado
- 1 cup strawberries
- 6-8 oz. coconut water + 6-8 ounces of filtered water
- Fresh juice of one lime
- 1-2 teaspoon olive oil

Directions:

1. Add listed ingredients to a blender
2. Blend until you have a smooth and creamy texture

3. Serve chilled and enjoy!

Nutrition:
Calories: 409, Fat: 33 g, Carbs: 8 g, Protein: 12 g
264. Ginger Strawberry Shake
Preparation Time: 10 minutes
Cooking Time: 0 minutes
Servings: 1
Ingredients:

- 1 cup almond milk
- ½ teaspoon ginger powder
- 1 small stalk celery
- 1 cup spring salad mix
- 1 teaspoon sesame seeds
- 1 cup of water
- 1 pack Stevia

Directions:

1. Add listed ingredients to a blender
2. Blend until you have a smooth and creamy texture
3. Serve chilled and enjoy!

Nutrition:
Calories: 475, Fat: 50 g, Carbs: 10 g, Protein: 7 g
265. Almond and Kale Extreme
Preparation Time: 10 minutes
Cooking Time: 0 minutes
Servings: 1
Ingredients:

- ¼ cup kale, torn
- 2 cups of water
- 2-Oz almonds
- 1 packet Stevia, if desired
- ½ cup spinach, packed

Directions:

1. Soak almonds in water and keep it overnight.
2. Do not discard water and add it all in a blender.
3. Add all the listed ingredients to a blender.
4. Blend on high until smooth and creamy.
5. Enjoy your smoothie.

Nutrition:
Calories: 334, Fat: 28 g, Carbs: 14 g, Protein: 12 g
266. Berry Shake
Preparation Time: 10 minutes
Cooking Time: 0 minutes
Servings: 1
Ingredients:

- ½ cup whole milk yogurt
- ¼ cup raspberries
- ¼ cup blackberry
- ¼ cup strawberries, chopped
- 1 tablespoon cocoa powder
- 1 ½ cups of water

Directions:

1. Add listed ingredients to a blender
2. Blend until you have a smooth and creamy texture
3. Serve chilled and enjoy!

Nutrition:
Calories: 255, Fat: 19 g, Carbs: 20 g, Protein: 6 g
267. Watermelon Sorbet
Preparation Time: 20 minutes + 20 hours' chill time
Cooking Time: 0 minutes
Servings: 4
Ingredients:

- 4 cups watermelons, seedless and chunked
- ¼ cup of coconut sugar
- 2 tablespoons of lime juice

Directions:

1. Add the listed ingredients to a blender and puree
2. Transfer to a freezer container with a tight-fitting lid
3. Freeze the mix for about 4-6 hours until you have gelatin-like consistency
4. Puree the mix once again in batches and return to the container
5. Chill overnight
6. Allow the sorbet to stand for 5 minutes before Servings: and enjoy!

Nutrition:
Calories: 91, Carbs: 25 g, Protein: 1 g

268. Berry Smoothie
Preparation Time: 4 minutes
Cooking Time: 0 minutes
Servings: 2
Ingredients:

- ¼ cup of frozen blueberries
- ¼ cup of frozen blackberries
- 1 cup of unsweetened almond milk
- 1 teaspoon of vanilla bean extract
- 3 teaspoons of flaxseed
- 1 scoop of chilled Greek yogurt
- Stevia as needed

Directions:

1. Mix everything in a blender and emulsify.
2. Pulse the mixture four-times until you have your desired thickness.
3. Pour the mixture into a glass and enjoy!

Nutrition:
Calories: 221, Fat: 9 g, Protein: 21 g, Carbs: 10 g

269. Berry and Almond Smoothie
Preparation Time: 10 minutes
Cooking Time: nil

Servings: 4
Ingredients:

- 1 cup of blueberries, frozen
- 1 whole banana
- ½ a cup of almond milk
- 1 tablespoon of almond butter
- Water as needed

Directions:

1. Add the listed ingredients to your blender and blend well until you have a smoothie-like texture
2. Chill and serve
3. Enjoy!

Nutrition:
Calories: 321, Fat: 11 g, Carbs: 55 g, Protein: 5 g

270. Mango and Pear Smoothie
Preparation Time: 10 minutes
Cooking Time: Nil
Servings: 1
Ingredients:

- 1 ripe mango, cored and chopped
- ½ mango, peeled, pitted, and chopped
- 1 cup kale, chopped
- ½ cup plain Greek yogurt
- 2 ice cubes

Directions:

1. Add pear, mango, yogurt, kale, and mango to a blender and puree
2. Add ice and blend until you have a smooth texture
3. Serve and enjoy!

Nutrition:
Calories: 293, Fat: 8 g, Carbs: 53 g, Protein: 8 g

271. Pineapple Juice
Preparation Time: 10 minutes
Cooking Time: nil
Servings: 4
Ingredients:

- 4 cups of fresh pineapple, chopped
- 1 pinch of sunflower seeds
- 1 ½ cup of water

Directions:

1. Add the listed ingredients to your blender and blend well until you have a smoothie-like texture
2. Chill and serve
3. Enjoy!

Nutrition:
Calories: 82, Fat: 0.2 g, Carbs: 21 g, Protein: 21 g
272. Coffee Smoothie
Preparation Time: 10 minutes
Cooking Time: 0 minutes
Servings: 1
Ingredients:

- 1 tablespoon chia seeds
- 2 cups strongly brewed coffee, chilled
- 1-ounce Macadamia nuts
- 1-2 packets Stevia, optional
- 1 tablespoon MCT oil

Directions:

1. Add all the listed ingredients to a blender
2. Blend on high until smooth and creamy
3. Enjoy your smoothie

Nutrition:
Calories: 395, Fat: 39 g, Carbs: 11 g, Protein: 5.2 g

273. Blackberry and Apple Smoothie
Preparation Time: 5 minutes
Cooking Time: 0 minutes
Servings: 2
Ingredients:

- 2 cups frozen blackberries
- ½ cup apple cider
- 1 apple, cubed
- ⅔ cup nonfat lemon yogurt

Directions:

1. Add the listed ingredients to your blender and blend until smooth
2. Serve chilled!

Nutrition:
Calories: 200, Fat: 10 g, Carbs: 14 g, Protein 2 g

274. Minty Cherry Smoothie
Preparation Time: 5 minutes
Cooking Time: 0 minutes
Servings: 2
Ingredients:

- ¾ cup cherries
- 1 teaspoon minutest
- ½ cup almond milk
- ½ cup kale
- ½ teaspoon fresh vanilla

Directions:

1. Wash and cut cherries
2. Take the pits out
3. Add cherries to the blender
4. Pour almond milk
5. Wash the minutest and put two sprigs in blender
6. Separate the kale leaves from the stems

7. Put kale in a blender
8. Press vanilla bean and cut lengthwise with a knife
9. Scoop out your desired amount of vanilla and add to the blender
10. Blend until smooth
11. Serve chilled and enjoy!

Nutrition:
Calories: 200, Fat: 10 g, Carbs: 14 g, Protein 2 g

275. Fruit Smoothie
Preparation Time: 10 minutes
Cooking Time: 0 minutes
Servings: 1
Ingredients:

- 1 cup spring mix salad blend
- 2 cups of water
- 3 medium blackberries, whole
- 1 packet Stevia, optional
- 1 tablespoon coconut flakes shredded and unsweetened
- 2 tablespoons pecans, chopped
- 1 tablespoon hemp seed
- 1 tablespoon sunflower seed

Directions:

1. Add all the listed ingredients to a blender
2. Blend on high until smooth and creamy
3. Enjoy your smoothie

Nutrition:
Calories: 385, Fat: 34 g, Carbs: 16 g, Protein: 6.9 g

276. Blueberry Blast Smoothie
Preparation Time: 10 minutes
Cooking Time: 0 minutes
Servings: 1
Ingredients:
- 1 cup frozen blueberries
- 8 packets of Splenda

- 6 tbsp. of protein powder
- 8 ice cubes
- 14 oz. apple juice

Directions:

1. Put all the ingredients in the blender.
2. Give it a pulse for 30 seconds until blended well.
3. Serve chilled and fresh.

Nutrition:
Calories: 108, Protein: 9 g, Carbs: 18 g, Fat: 0.2 g, Cholesterol: 0.01 mg, Sodium: 27 mg, Potassium: 183 mg, Phosphorus: 42 mg, Calcium: 57 mg, Fiber: 1.2 g

277. Pineapple Protein Smoothie
Preparation Time: 10 minutes
Cooking Time: 0 minutes
Servings: 1
Ingredients:

- ¾ cup pineapple sorbet
- 1 scoop vanilla protein powder
- ½ cup water
- 2 ice cubes, optional

Directions:

1. Put all the ingredients in the blender.
2. Give it a pulse for 30 seconds until blended well.
3. Serve chilled and fresh.

Nutrition:
Calories: 268, Protein: 18 g, Carbs: 40 g, Fat: 4 g, Cholesterol: 36 mg, Sodium: 93 mg, Potassium: 237 mg, Phosphorus: 160 mg, Calcium: 160 mg, Fiber: 1.4 g

278. Fruity Smoothie
Preparation Time: 10 minutes
Cooking Time: 0 minutes
Servings: 2
Ingredients:

- 8 oz. canned fruits, with juice
- 2 scoops vanilla-flavored whey protein powder

- 1 cup cold water
- 1 cup crushed ice

Directions:

1. Put all the ingredients in the blender.
2. Give it a pulse for 30 seconds until blended well.
3. Serve chilled and fresh.

Nutrition:
Calories: 186, Protein: 23 g, Carbs: 19 g, Fat: 2 g, Cholesterol: 41 mg, Sodium: 62 mg, Potassium: 282 mg, Phosphorus: 118 mg, Calcium: 160 mg, Fiber: 1.1 g

279. Mixed Berry Protein Smoothie
Preparation Time: 10 minutes
Cooking Time: 0 minutes
Servings: 2
Ingredients:

- 4 oz. cold water
- 1 cup frozen mixed berries
- 2 ice cubes
- 1 tsp blueberry essence
- ½ cup whipped cream topping
- 2 scoops whey protein powder

Directions:

1. Put all the ingredients in the blender.
2. Give it a pulse for 30 seconds until blended well.
3. Serve chilled and fresh.

Nutrition:
Calories: 104, Protein: 6 g, Carbs: 11 g, Fat: 4 g, Cholesterol: 11 mg, Sodium: 15 mg, Potassium: 141 mg, Phosphorus: 49 mg, Calcium: 69 mg, Fiber: 2.4 g

280. Peach High-Protein Smoothie
Preparation Time: 10 minutes
Cooking Time: 0 minutes
Servings: 1
Ingredients:

- ½ cup ice

- 2 tbsp. powdered egg whites
- ¾ cup fresh peaches
- 1 tbsp. sugar

Directions:

1. Put all the ingredients in the blender.
2. Give it a pulse for 30 seconds until blended well.
3. Serve chilled and fresh.

Nutrition:
Calories: 132, Protein: 10 g, Carbs: 24 g, Sodium: 154 mg, Potassium: 353 mg, Phosphorus: 36 mg, Calcium: 9 mg, Fiber: 1.9 g

281. Strawberry Fruit Smoothie
Preparation Time: 10 minutes
Cooking Time: 0 minutes
Servings: 1
Ingredients:
- ¾ cup fresh strawberries
- ½ cup liquid pasteurized egg whites
- ½ cup ice
- 1 tbsp. sugar

Directions:

1. Put all the ingredients in the blender.
2. Give it a pulse for 30 seconds until blended well.
3. Serve chilled and fresh.

Nutrition:
Calories: 156, Protein: 14 g, Carbs: 25 g, Sodium: 215 mg, Potassium: 400 mg, Phosphorus: 49 mg, Calcium: 29 mg, Fiber: 2.5 g

282. Watermelon Bliss
Preparation time: 10 minutes
Cooking time: 0 minutes
Servings: 2
Ingredients:
- 2 cups watermelon
- 1 medium-sized cucumber, peeled and sliced
- 2 mint sprigs, leaves only
- 1 celery stalk

- A squeeze of lime juice

Directions:

1. Put all the ingredients in the blender.
2. Give it a pulse for 30 seconds until blended well.
3. Serve chilled and fresh.

Nutrition:
Calories: 156, Protein: 14 g, Carbs: 25 g, Sodium: 215 mg, Potassium: 400 mg, Phosphorus: 49 mg, Calcium: 29 mg, Fiber: 2.5 g

283. Cranberry Smoothie
Preparation Time: 10 minutes
Cooking Time: 0 minutes
Servings: 1
Ingredients:
- 1 cup frozen cranberries
- 1 medium cucumber, peeled and sliced
- 1 stalk of celery
- Handful of parsley
- A squeeze of lime juice

Directions:

1. Put all the ingredients in the blender.
2. Give it a pulse for 30 seconds until blended well.
3. Serve chilled and fresh.

Nutrition:
Calories: 126, Protein: 12 g, Carbs: 35 g, Fat: 0.03 g, Sodium: 125 mg, Potassium: 220 mg, Phosphorus: 219 mg, Calcium: 19 mg, Fiber: 1.4 g

284. Berry Cucumber Smoothie
Preparation Time: 10 minutes
Cooking Time: 0 minutes
Servings: 1
Ingredients:
- 1 medium cucumber, peeled and sliced
- ½ cup fresh blueberries
- ½ cup fresh or frozen strawberries
- ½ cup unsweetened rice milk
- Stevia, to taste

Directions:

1. Put all the ingredients in the blender.
2. Give it a pulse for 30 seconds until blended well.
3. Serve chilled and fresh.

Nutrition:
Calories: 141, Protein: 10 g, Carbs: 15 g, Sodium: 113 mg, Potassium: 230 mg, Phosphorus: 129 mg, Calcium: 15 mg, Fiber: 3.1 g

285. Raspberry Peach Smoothie
Preparation time: 10 minutes
Cooking time: 0 minutes
Servings: 2
Ingredients:
- 1 cup frozen raspberries
- 1 medium peach, pit removed, sliced
- ½ cup silken tofu
- 1 tbsp. honey
- 1 cup unsweetened vanilla almond milk

Directions:

1. Put all the ingredients in the blender.
2. Give it a pulse for 30 seconds until blended well.
3. Serve chilled and fresh.

Nutrition:
Calories: 132, Protein: 9 g, Carbs: 14 g, Sodium: 112 mg, Potassium: 310 mg, Phosphorus: 39 mg, Calcium: 32 mg, Fiber: 1.4 g

Recipes for Kids

286. Blackberry Pudding
Preparation Time: 45 minutes
Cooking Time: 0
Servings: 2
Ingredients:
- ¼ cup chia seeds
- ½ cup blackberries, fresh
- 1 tsp. liquid sweetener

- 1 cup coconut milk, full fat and unsweetened
- 1 tsp. vanilla extract

Directions:

1. Take the vanilla, liquid sweetener, and coconut milk and add to the blender
2. Process until thick
3. Add blackberries and process until smooth
4. Divide the mixture between cups and chill for 30 minutes
5. Serve and enjoy!

Nutrition:
Calories: 437, Fat: 38 g, Carbs: 8 g, Protein: 8 g

287. Simple Green Shake
Preparation Time: 10 minutes
Cooking Time: 0
Servings: 1
Ingredients:

- ¾ cup whole milk yogurt
- 2½ cups lettuce, mix salad greens
- 1 pack stevia
- 1 tbsp. MCT oil
- 1 tbsp. chia seeds
- 1 ½ cups of water

Directions:

1. Add listed ingredients to a blender
2. Blend until you have a smooth and creamy texture
3. Serve chilled and enjoy!

Nutrition:
Calories: 320, Fat: 24 g, Carbs: 17 g, Protein: 10 g

288. Green Beans and Roasted Onion
Preparation Time: 10 minutes
Cooking Time: 15 minutes
Servings: 6
Ingredients:

- 1 yellow onion, sliced into rings
- ½ tsp. onion powder

- 2 tbsps. coconut flour
- 1 ⅓ pound fresh green beans, trimmed and chopped
- ½ tbsp. salt

Directions:

1. Take a large bowl and mix the salt with the onion powder and coconut flour
2. Add onion rings
3. Mix well to coat
4. Spread the rings in the baking sheet, lined with parchment paper
5. Drizzle with some oil
6. Bake for 10 minutes at 400°F
7. Parboil the green beans for 3 to 5 minutes in the boiling water
8. Drain and serve the beans with the baked onion rings
9. Serve warm and enjoy!

Nutrition:
Calories: 214, Fat: 19.4 g, Carbs: 3.7 g, Protein: 8.3 g

289. Zucchini and Onion Platter
Preparation Time: 15 minutes
Cooking Time: 45 minutes
Servings: 4
Ingredients:

- 3 large zucchinis, julienned
- ½ cup basil
- 2 red onions, thinly sliced
- ¼ tsp. salt
- 1 tsp. cayenne pepper
- 2 tbsps. lemon juice

Directions:

1. Create zucchini Zoodles by using a vegetable peeler and shaving the zucchini with the peeler lengthwise until you get to the core and seeds
2. Turn zucchini and repeat until you have long strips
3. Discard seeds
4. Lay strips on cutting board and slice lengthwise to your desired thickness

5. Mix Zoodles in a bowl alongside onion, basil, and toss
6. Sprinkle salt and cayenne pepper on top
7. Drizzle lemon juice

Nutrition:
Calories: 156, Fat: 8 g, Carbs: 6 g, Protein: 7 g

290. Onion Cheese Omelet
Preparation Time: 3 minutes
Cooking Time: 12 minutes
Servings: 2
Ingredients:
- 3 eggs
- ¼ cup liquid creamer
- 1 tbsp. water
- Black pepper to taste
- 1 tbsp. butter
- ¾cup onion, sliced
- 1 large apple, peeled, cored, and sliced
- 2 tbsps. Cheddar cheese, grated

Directions:

1. Preheat the oven to 400 degrees F.
2. Whisk the eggs with the liquid creamer, water, and black pepper in a suitable bowl.
3. Stir ¼ of the butter into an oven-safe skillet and sauté the onion and apple slices.
4. After 5 minutes, pour in the egg mixture over the onions.
5. Sprinkle Cheddar cheese over the egg and bake for 12 minutes. Slice the omelet and serve.

Nutrition:
Calories: 254, Fat: 15.1 g, Cholesterol: 268 mg, Sodium: 184 mg, Carbs: 20.7 g, Fiber: 3.6 g, Sugars: 14.6 g, Protein: 10.9 g, Calcium: 98 mg, Phosphorous: 334 mg, Potassium: 280 mg

291. Morning Patties
Preparation Time: 3 minutes
Cooking Time: 6 minutes
Servings: 6
Ingredients:

- 1 lb. fresh lean ground chicken
- 2 tsps. ground sage
- 2 tsps. granulated Swerve
- 1 tsp. ground black pepper
- ½ tsp. ground red pepper
- 1 tsp. basil

Directions:

1. Mix the ground chicken with the sage, Swerve, black pepper, red pepper, and basil in a suitable bowl.
2. Take 2 tbsps. of this meat mixture and make a patty.
3. Grease a cooking pan with cooking spray and place it over moderate heat.
4. Add the patties to the pan and sear them for 2-3 minutes per side.
5. Optional: Serve with fresh bread.

Nutrition:
Calories: 115, Fat: 6.2 g, Cholesterol: 65 mg, Sodium: 46 mg, Carbs: 0.8 g, Fiber: 0.2 g, Sugars: 0.3 g, Protein: 13.3 g Calcium: 10 mg, Phosphorous: 200 mg, Potassium: 405 mg

292. Mushroom Omelet
Preparation Time: 3 minutes
Cooking Time: 10 minutes
Servings: 2
Ingredients:

- 2 tbsps. and 1 tsp. olive oil
- 1 shallot, minced
- ¼ lb. cremini mushrooms, rinsed
- Black pepper to taste
- 1 garlic clove, minced
- 2 tsps. parsley, minced
- 4 eggs
- 1 tbsp. chives, minced
- 2 tsps. milk
- 3 tbsps. Gruyere cheese, grated

Directions:

1. Set a suitable non-stick skillet over moderate heat and add 1

tsp. olive oil.

2. Add in the shallot and mushrooms, then sauté for 5 minutes until soft.
3. Toss in the garlic and sauté for 1 minute.
4. Now add the rest of the oil to the same skillet.
5. Mix the eggs with the chives, milk, and black pepper in a bowl and pour it into the skillet.
6. Cook the egg omelet for about 2 minutes per side until golden brown then transfers to the serving place.
7. Serve with Gruyere cheese and parsley on top.

Nutrition:
Calories: 271, Fat: 23 g, Cholesterol: 328 mg, Sodium: 208 mg, Carbs: 4.8 g, Fiber: 0.5 g, Sugars: 2 g, Protein: 13 g, Calcium: 71 mg, Phosphorous: 227 mg, Potassium: 410 mg

293. Garlicky Balsamic Chicken
Preparation Time: 3 minutes
Cooking Time: 30 minutes
Servings: 8
Ingredients:
- 2 cups low-sodium chicken broth
- ½ cup balsamic vinegar
- ½ cup white wine
- 1 tbsp., rosemary, chopped
- 8 chicken breasts, boneless, skinless
- 1 garlic head, chopped
- 2 tbsps. olive oil
- Black pepper, to taste

Directions:

1. Begin by mixing the wine, rosemary, broth, and vinegar in a 9x13 inch baking pan.
2. Add the chicken breasts and rub well with the mixture. Marinate overnight.
3. Grease a saucepan with oil and add the garlic.
4. Sauté until golden, then keep the garlic aside.
5. Season the marinated chicken with black pepper and sear it for 5 minutes per side until golden.
6. Pour the reserved marinade over it along with the garlic.

7. Cook on reduced heat for 15 minutes and flip the chicken after 7 minutes.
8. Transfer the chicken to the serving plates.
9. Cook the remaining cooking liquid until it thickens.
10. Pour the sauce over the chicken.
11. Serve warm and fresh.

Nutrition:
Calories: 265, Fat: 3.4 g, Cholesterol: 130 mg, Sodium: 188 mg, Carbs: 1.6 g, Fiber: 0.3 g, Sugars: 0.2 g, Protein: 37.3 g, Calcium: 11 mg, Phosphorous: 221 mg, Potassium: 34 mg

294. Salisbury Meat Steak
Preparation Time: 5 minutes
Cooking Time: 25 minutes
Servings: 4
Ingredients:
- 1 lb. steak, finely chopped
- 1 small onion, chopped
- ½ cup green pepper, chopped
- 1 tsp. black pepper
- 1 egg
- 1 tbsp. olive oil
- ½ cup water
- 1 tbsp. corn starch

Directions:

1. Mix the steak with the green pepper, egg, black pepper, and onion in a bowl.
2. Add the oil to a skillet and place the patties in.
3. Sear the steak patties for 5 minutes per side until golden brown.
4. Add half of the water and let the patties simmer for 15 minutes.
5. Whisk the remaining water with cornstarch in a bowl.
6. Add this cornstarch mixture to the patties and cook until the sauce thickens.
7. Serve warm.

Nutrition:
Calories: 276, Fat: 11.6 g, Cholesterol: 142 mg, Sodium: 92 mg, Carbs:

4.8 g, Fiber: 0.7 g, Sugars: 1.1 g, Protein: 33.1 g, Calcium: 16 mg, Phosphorous: 361 mg, Potassium: 524 mg

295. Eggplant Fries
Preparation time: 10 minutes
Cooking Time: 5 minutes
Servings: 6
Ingredients:

- 2 eggs, beaten
- 1 cup almond milk
- 1 tsp. hot sauce
- ¾ cup cornstarch
- 3 tsps. dry ranch seasoning mix
- ¾ cup dry breadcrumbs
- 1 eggplant, sliced into strips
- ½ cup oil

Directions:

1. In a bowl, mix eggs, milk, and hot sauce.
2. In a dish, mix cornstarch, seasoning, and breadcrumbs.
3. Dip first the eggplant strips in the egg mixture.
4. Coat each strip with the cornstarch mixture.
5. Pour oil into a pan over medium heat.
6. Once hot, add the fries and cook for 3 minutes or until golden.

Nutrition:

Calories: 233, Protein: 5 g, Carbs: 24 g, Fat: 13 g, Cholesterol: 48 mg, Sodium: 212 mg, Potassium: 215 mg, Phosphorus: 86 mg, Calcium: 70 mg, Fiber: 2.1 g

296. Seasoned Green Beans
Preparation Time: 10 minutes
Cooking Time: 10 minutes
Servings: 4
Ingredients:

- 10 oz. green beans
- 4 tsps. butter
- ¼ cup onion, chopped
- ½ cup red bell pepper, chopped
- 1 tsp. dried dill weed
- 1 tsp. dried parsley

- ¼ tsp. black pepper

Directions:

1. Boil green beans in a pot of water. Drain.
2. In a pan over medium heat, melt the butter and cook onion and bell pepper.
3. Season with dill and parsley.
4. Put the green beans back to the skillet.
5. Sprinkle pepper on top before serving.

Nutrition:
Calories: 67, Protein: 2 g, Carbs: 8 g, Fat: 3 g, Sodium: 55 mg, Potassium: 194 mg, Phosphorus: 32 mg, Calcium: 68 mg, Fiber: 4.0 g

297. Grilled Squash
Preparation Time: 10 minutes
Cooking Time: 6 minutes
Servings: 8
Ingredients:
- 4 zucchinis, rinsed, drained, and sliced
- 4 crookneck squash, rinsed, drained, and sliced
- Cooking spray
- ¼ tsp. garlic powder
- ¼ tsp. black pepper

Directions:

1. Arrange squash on a baking sheet.
2. Spray with oil.
3. Season with garlic powder and pepper.
4. Grill for 3 minutes per side or until tender but not too soft.

Nutrition:
Calories: 17, Protein: 1 g, Carbs: 3 g, Sodium: 6 mg, Potassium: 262 mg, Phosphorus: 39 mg, Calcium: 16 mg, Fiber: 1.1 g

AFTERWORD

Yes, although your metabolism is generally fairly stable, you can do several things to help rev it up.

No. 1 is exercise.

Working out creates muscles. Metabolism speeds up the muscles. It processes food faster as the body works more effectively, and your appetite increases. That's why my bodybuilding client had trouble controlling his hunger.

Men generally burn more calories than a woman of the same weight, being the more muscular sex. This is why the law student was having a harder time than her husband losing the weight.

Don't overlook meals.

Meals should take in space, 3-4 hours apart. That way, throughout the day, you have enough energy, and you will be free from the headaches, hunger pangs, or mood swings that you get when you're hungry.

The body is erratically signaled to burn slower and preserve fat by eating. This is why, 1,200 calories, the law student who skipped meals does not lose weight. Throughout the day, she would be best off having smaller, balanced meals and snacks.

A balanced nutrition and exercise plan, which promotes an average weight loss rate of 1-2 pounds per week, it is the way to lose more fat than muscle.

Food influences the mood.

Your metabolism and mood are affected by what you eat, making you either sluggish or energized. Foods that are high in sugar, saturated fats, artificial sweeteners, low in water and fiber it can slow your digestion, cause weight gain, and make you feel like a couch potato.

The proteins, carbohydrates, and fats that give you energy and even blood sugar levels are supplied by whole grains, vegetables, fruits, beans, legumes, fresh herbs and spices. Long-lasting, stable energy levels are promoted by healthy fats (olive oil, avocado, fish oils, seeds, nuts, soybeans). For better digestion and muscle building, lean proteins (fish, soy foods, white meat poultry, lean meats and low-fat dairy) offer essential proteins.

You will have better digestion by drinking eight glasses of water everyday (better emptying of the stomach and intestines, less gas, bloating, constipation) and a flatter stomach. Staying hydrated also decreases fatigue from headaches and fights.

You ought to get pleasure from eating too. Even if it is your wish to add a piece of dark chocolate, go for it, one square at a time, as it helps with the happy brain chemistry and adds a natural bitter that helps digestion. This way, improving digestion also strengthens the liver, kidneys and lungs, all of which make a healthier metabolism easier.

Stay Cool

In order to keep the body warm, in a colder weather it increases metabolism, although maintaining your weight during the holidays and colder months can be a challenge when exercise levels tend to drop, and pounds often pile on.

You can burn more calories by keeping indoor temperatures coolers and exercising outdoors.

You'll feel more energetic, lighter, and hungrier as your metabolism increases. But don't be afraid. The stomach empties more regularly as digestion improves, and you feel thinner in the waistline and less full in the chest. People with a faster metabolism have fewer cravings for food and they feel more to control of their consumption.

Don't get trapped in a rut.

At a certain weight, some dieters get stuck. You must make small changes to keep your body from adapting to a routine of eating the same amount of calories to keep your weight from plateauing.

If you can't lose those last five pounds, add two weeks of a few hundred more calories a day, and then return to a smaller amount. This approach will allow you to boost the number of calories you can eat over the time and continue to lose weight.

Have patience

Increasing your metabolism may take you some time like three months is a reasonable timeframe to expect to see the changes. You might consider having your metabolism tested by a professional nutritionist if you are having a hard time to lose weight.

Being persistent, having trust and being patient is the key.

You will feel healthier and stronger soon, and the results of a toned, healthier body will be seen in time. Best of all, you're going to have a more clear understanding of what makes your body feel and work better, so for years to come, you'll be able to control your weight more effectively.

This way, results were achieved by the both my law student and bodybuilder clients.

The lawyer was given an increased, longer-lasting energy level by a regular routine of having easy meals and snacks on hand and spreading her calorie intake throughout the day.

And by eating more regular, balanced meals and incorporating whole grain, fruits, vegetables and healthy fats into his snacking routine, the bodybuilder have lost the weight.

The Best Foods for Improving Your Metabolism

Your metabolism can be increased by the certain foods.

The more calories you burn, the higher your metabolism gets, and the easier it is to maintain your weight or get rid of unwanted body fat.

Here are 12 foods that can help you to lose weight by boosting your metabolism.

1. Protein-Rich Foods

For a few hours, protein-rich foods such as meat, fish, eggs, dairy, legumes, nuts, and seeds can help to boost your metabolism.

By requiring your body to use additional energy to digest them, they do so.

This is known as the Food Thermal Effect (TEF). TEF refers to the number of calories that your body needs in your meals to digest, absorb and process the nutrients.

Protein-rich foods increase TEF the most, research shows. They boost your metabolic rate, for instance, by 15-30 percent, compared to 5-10 percent for carbs and 0-3 percent for fats. By helping your body keep its muscle mass, protein-rich diets also reduce the drop in metabolism often seen during the weight loss. Moreover, protein can also help to keep you fuller for longer, which can also stop overeating.

2. Iron, Zinc, and Selenium-Rich Foods Rich

In the proper function of your body, iron, zinc and selenium each play distinct but equally significant roles.

They do have one thing in common; however: all three are necessary for the proper function of your thyroid gland, which controls your metabolism. Research shows that a diet that is too low in iron, zinc or selenium may decrease your thyroid gland's ability to produce enough hormones. This can make your metabolism slow down. In order to help to get your thyroid function to the best of its ability, your daily menu includes zinc, selenium and iron-rich foods such as meat, seafood, legumes, nuts and seeds.

3. Chili Peppers

By increasing the amount of calories and fat you burn, capsaicin, a chemical found in chili peppers, may boost your metabolism.

A review of 20 research studies actually reports that capsaicin can help your body to burn about 50 extra calories a day. After intake of 135-150 mg of capsaicin per day, this effect was initially observed, but some studies reported similar benefits with doses as low as 9-10 mg per day. Capsaicin may, in addition, have appetite-reducing properties.

According to a study, it shows that consuming 2 mg of capsaicin directly before each meal reduces the number of calories which is consumed, particularly from carbohydrates.

4. Coffee

Studies report that up to 11 percent of the caffeine found in the coffee can help to increase the metabolic rate. Six different studies have actually found that people who consume at least 270 mg of caffeine a day, or about three cups of coffee, burn an additional 100 calories a day. In addition, caffeine can also help your body to burn fat for energy and it seems particularly effective at boosting the performance of your workout. However, its effects, based on individual characteristics such as body weight and age, seem to vary from person to person.

5. Tea

The mixture of caffeine and catechins found in tea may work to boost your metabolism, according to research.

Both oolong and green tea can improve metabolism by 4-10 percent in particular. This might add up to an extra 100 calories per day being burned. In addition, oolong and green teas can help your body more effectively to use stored fat for energy, increasing your capacity to burn fat by up to 17 percent. Nonetheless, as is the case with coffee, effects can differ from individual to individual.

6. Pulses and Legumes

In comparison to other plant foods, legumes and pulses, such as lentils, peas, chickpeas, beans and peanuts, are particularly high in protein.

Studies suggest that, compared to lower-protein foods, their high protein content requires your body to burn a greater number of calories to digest them. Legumes also contain a good quantity of dietary fiber that your body can use to feed the good bacteria living in your intestines, such as resistant starch and soluble fiber. These friendly bacteria, in turn, generate short-chain fatty acids that can help your body to use stored fat as an energy and maintain normal levels of the blood sugar. In one study, individuals eating a diet rich in legumes for eight weeks may experience beneficial metabolic changes and lost 1.5 times more weight than the control group. Arginine, an amino acid that might increase the amount of carbs and fat in your body can burn for energy, it is also high in legumes.

There are also substantial amounts of amino acid glutamine in peas, fava beans and lentils, which can help to increase the number of calories burned during digestion.

7. Metabolism-Boosting Spices

It is thought that certain spices have particularly beneficial metabolism-boosting properties.

Research shows, for example, that dissolving 2 grams of ginger powder in the hot water and drinking it with food can help you to burn up to 43 more calories than drinking hot water alone. This hot ginger drink also appears to decrease the hunger levels and improve feelings of satiety. Grains of paradise, another of the ginger family's spices, can also have similar the effects.

A recent study reported that in the following two hours, participants given a 40-mg extract of Paradise grains burned 43 more calories than those who were given a placebo. Researchers also noted that non-responders are part of the participants, so the effects can vary from one person to another.

Similarly, adding cayenne pepper to your meal, particularly after a high-fat meal, may increase the amount of fat in your body that burns for energy. This fat-burning effect, however, may only apply to individuals unaccustomed to eat spicy foods.

8. Cacao

Cacao and cocoa are delicious treats that might benefit your metabolism as well.

Studies in mice, for instance, have found that cocoa and cocoa extracts may promote gene expression that stimulates the use of fat for the energy. In mice fed high-fat or high-calorie diets, this seems particularly true. Interestingly, one study suggests that the action of enzymes necessary to break down the fat and carbs during digestion may be prevented by cocoa. In doing so, by reducing the absorption of some calories, cocoa could theoretically play a part in preventing weight gain.

Human studies investigating the effects of cocoa, cacao or cacao products such as dark chocolate, however, are uncommon. Before strong conclusions can be made, more studies are required. If you want to try cacao, opt for raw versions, as the quantities of beneficial compounds tend to be reduced by the processing.

9. Apple Cider Vinegar

Your metabolism can also be increased by apple cider vinegar.

Vinegar has been shown by several animal studies to be particularly helpful in increasing the amount of fat burned for energy.

Mice given vinegar had an increase in the enzyme AMPK in one of the study, which prompts the body to reduce fat storage and increase fat burning.

In another study, vinegar-treated obese rats experienced an increase in the expression of certain genes, leading to a decreased storage of liver fat and belly fat. Apple cider vinegar is often claimed to increase human metabolism, but few studies have directly investigated the matter.

Apple cider vinegar, however, may still help you to lose weight in other ways, such as slowing the emptying of the stomach and improving feelings of fullness.

One human study even showed that respondents who were given four teaspoons (20 ml) of apple cider vinegar ate up to 275 fewer calories during the rest of the day. Be careful to limit your daily intake to two tablespoons (30 ml) if you would like to give apple cider vinegar a try.

We have the wrong weight loss ideas, which at best makes the whole process difficult and it simply do not work at worst. Since most individuals do not need weight-loss experts, they do not see this and they follow the old methods, such as lemmings, in the hope that they can lose the weight.

We've got it all wrong about losing the weight. Food restriction and deprivation mixed with the excessive amounts of repetitive low-intensity activity are included in the old accepted but not workable path to weight loss. These old-fashioned strategies that cause mental conflict and physical suffering and are not enjoyed by most people and don't give us the weight loss we want anyway.

Not all, but a great percentage of people have gained weight from a long-term hormonal balance, many of them are women. This can be caused by the repeated dieting, insufficient muscular exertion and excessive activity of the 'cardio' type. For those people, who are trying to lose weight again will exacerbate the problem and make it almost impossible to achieve the goal of long-term weight loss. It is in a poor state with fat storage/fat-burning hormones 'out of whack' when the human body becomes overweight (over fat). Restricting the intake of food and too much of the wrong type of exercise does not solve the issue.

In fact, it makes us unhealthier because those things work against the body, causing an inefficient metabolism (the engine of the body) that is even slower. By day and night, it reduces the amount of fuel (calories) that we burn, and this is how we get and stay overweight. Only when the body system is strong and healthy weight loss can be happen. It takes a shift both mentally and physically to take the body from an unhealthy state to better 'metabolic fitness' before weight loss can occur, so it can burn fat for the energy and not to store it.

In this book, we have discussed that how, with the Octavia diet, you could maintain a good long-term relationship with food, reset your metabolism and achieve the desired weight loss.

You likely had little knowledge about your kidneys before. You probably didn't know how you could take steps to improve the health of your kidneys and decrease the risk of developing kidney failure. However, through reading this book, you now understand the power of the human kidney, as well as the prognosis of Chronic Kidney Disease.

In general, your body converts several things that appear to be benign until the body's organs convert them to things like formaldehyde, due to a synthetic response and transformation phase. One such case is a large part of the dietary sugars used in diet sodas—for example, aspartame is converted to formaldehyde in the body. These toxins must be excreted, or they can cause disease, renal (kidney) failure, malignant growth, and various other painful problems

Renal failure isn't a condition that occurs without any anticipation. It is a dynamic issue that may be found early and treated. It's conceivable to have partial renal failure, though it requires some time, or downright poor diet for a short time, to arrive at absolute renal failure. You would prefer not to reach total renal failure since this will require standard dialysis treatments to save your life. Dialysis treatments explicitly clean the blood of waste and toxins using a machine since your body can no longer carry out the responsibility. Without treatments, you could die a very painful death. Renal failure can be the consequence of long-haul diabetes, hypertension, unreliable diet, and can stem from other health concerns.

As for your well-being and health, it's a good idea to see your doctor as often as possible to make sure you don't have any issues that can easily be prevented. The kidneys are your body's channel from toxins (as is the liver). The moment you eat without control or drink liquor, you fill your body with toxins. Your kidneys clean the blood of unknown substances and remove toxins from things like preservatives in food.

While over thirty-million Americans are being affected by kidney disease, now you can take steps to be one of the people actively working to promote the health of your kidneys. These stats are alarming, which is why it is necessary to take proper care of your kidneys, starting with a kidney-friendly diet.

The recipes in the Renal Diet are ideal whether you have been diagnosed with a kidney problem or want to prevent any kidney issue. It is tied with directing the intake of protein and phosphorus in your eating routine. Restricting your sodium intake is likewise significant. By controlling these two variables, you can control most of the toxins and waste made by your body, and thus, this enables your kidney to function perfectly. If you catch onto renal failure early and truly moderate your diets with extraordinary consideration, you could avert the issue altogether.

www.ingramcontent.com/pod-product-compliance
Lightning Source LLC
Chambersburg PA
CBHW070901030426
42336CB00014BA/2278